Clinical Cases
for the MRCS
and AFRCS

Gareth J Morris-Stiff

MB, BCh, FRCS, is a Royal College of Surgeons Research Fellow in the Department of Surgery, University of Wales College of Medicine, Cardiff

David J Bowrey

MB, BCh, FRCS, is a Royal College of Surgeons Research Fellow in the Department of Surgery, University of Wales College of Medicine, Cardiff

Malcolm C A Puntis

MB, BCh, PhD, FRCS, is a Senior Lecturer in Surgery in the Department of Surgery, University of Wales College of Medicine, Cardiff and examiner for the MRCS

Brian I Rees

MA, MB, BChir, FRCS, is a Consultant Surgeon in the Department of Surgery, University Hospital of Wales, Cardiff, The Director of the Welsh Institute for Minimal Access Therapy (WIMAT) and examiner for the MRCS

Ahmed A Shandall

MB, BCh, MCh, FRCS, is a Consultant Surgeon in the Department of Surgery, Royal Gwent Hospital, Newport

A member of the Hodder Headline Group
LONDON
Distributed in the USA by Oxford University Press Inc., New York

E08184

First published in Great Britain in 1998
This impression printed in 2002 by
Arnold, a member of the Hodder Headline Group,
338 Euston Road, London NW1 3BH
http://www.arnoldpublishers.com

Distributed in the United States of America by
Oxford University Press Inc.,
198 Madison Avenue, New York, NY10016
Oxford is a registered trademark of Oxford University Press

British Library Cataloguing in Publication Data
A catalogue record for this book is available from the British Library

Library of Congress Cataloging-in-Publication Data
A catalog record for this book is available from the Library of Congress

ISBN 0 340 692 685 (pb)
3 4 5 6 7 8 9 10

Publisher: Annalisa Page
Production Editor: Rada Radojicic
Production Controller: Helen Whitehorn
Cover Design: Mouse Mat Design

Typeset in 9.5/12 pt Ocean Sans Light by
Scribe Design, Gillingham, Kent
Printed in Hong Kong

Contents

Foreword

The clinical part of the Fellowship examinations conducted by the four Royal Colleges of Surgeons has always been of special importance and, in particular, the 'short cases' have proved the downfall of many candidates. The new MRCS/AFRCS examinations also will lay great importance on the clinical part but the uncommon and unusual cases that were sometimes seen in the Fellowship will be excluded in favour of common surgical conditions ranged across all specialties. Despite the diminished experience as a result of shorter working hours and the shorter length of training required before sitting the examination, MRCS/AFRCS candidates will still need to acquire knowledge of the presentation and appearance of a wide spectrum of surgical conditions. It is my belief that this book will be of great help in this regard. Although it has been said that the greatest fool may ask more than the wisest man can answer, I firmly believe that candidates who have studied the illustrations and absorbed the text that follows this brief foreword will be well placed to impress their examiners. I join with the authors in wishing all candidates every success in their endeavours.

Barry Jackson, MS, FRCS
Chairman, Examinations Board,
Royal College of Surgeons of England
Member, Intercollegiate Committee in
Basic Surgical Training and Examinations

Preface

The recent changes in the format of the fellowship examinations have culminated in the introduction of the new MRCS and AFRCS examinations to replace the former FRCS. Despite these changes, however, clinical cases remain fundamental to the examinations. The ability to elicit an accurate history, to perform a clinical examination and implement the necessary intervention remains the essence of everyday surgical practice.

This book has been designed as an aid to the candidate preparing for the MRCS/AFRCS and concentrates on the commonly encountered aspects of general surgery and the more important aspects of other surgical specialties. In particular, the Orthopaedics and Trauma section affords an overview of the principles of treatment, rather than an exhaustive account of the management of the rarer conditions.

Each case scenario describes an actual patient history and follows in a systematic fashion the processes involved in obtaining a diagnosis to deciding upon the correct plan of management. The case selection is based upon the experiences of two of the authors who have recently been through the rigors of the FRCS together with advice from the remaining authors who are themselves college tutors or examiners.

We hope that candidates will find these cases to be an interesting and informative *aide memoire* during preparation for their surgical examinations and wish them the best of luck!

G.J.M-S.
D.J.B.
M.C.A.P.
B.I.R.
A.A.S.

Acknowledgements

We are indebted to the following for their assistance in the provision of clinical material or slide reproductions.

Dr M Allison, Consultant Gastroenterologist, Royal Gwent Hospital

Mr P D Carey, Senior Lecturer in Surgery, University Hospital of Wales

Mr G W B Clark, Lecturer in Surgery, University Hospital of Wales

Dr C J Davies, Consultant Radiologist, East Glamorgan Hospital

Mr W T Davies, Consultant Surgeon, University Hospital of Wales

Dr R J Evans, Consultant in Accident and Emergency, Cardiff Royal Infirmary

Mr M E Foster, Consultant Surgeon, East Glamorgan Hospital

Dr K Gower-Thomas, Consultant Radiologist, East Glamorgan Hospital

Dr D F Griffiths, Consultant Histopathologist, University Hospital of Wales

Dr K G Harding, Senior Lecturer in Wound Healing, University Hospital of Wales

Mr A J L Hart, Consultant Urologist, East Glamorgan Hospital

Dr E Hicks, Consultant Radiologist, East Glamorgan Hospital

Mr S Huddart, Consultant Paediatric Surgeon, University Hospital of Wales

Mr K Hutton, Consultant Paediatric Surgeon, University Hospital of Wales

Professor L E Hughes, Emeritus Professor of Surgery, University Hospital of Wales

Dr M Hourihan, Consultant Radiologist, University Hospital of Wales

Mr D A Jones, Surgical Senior House Officer, East Glamorgan Hospital

Mr D R Jones, Consultant Urologist, East Glamorgan Hospital

Mr W A Jurewicz, Consultant Transplant Surgeon, University Hospital of Wales

Mr I F Lane, Consultant Surgeon, University Hospital of Wales

Mr J Lari, Consultant Paediatric Surgeon, University Hospital of Wales

Miss R H H Lord, Consultant Transplant Surgeon, University Hospital of Wales

Professor R E Mansel, Professor of Surgery, University Hospital of Wales

Professor R Marks, Professor of Dermatology, University Hospital of Wales

Mr C Marnane, Surgical Senior House Officer, East Glamorgan Hospital

Mr R G S Mills, Consultant Ear, Nose and Throat Surgeon, University Hospital of Wales

Mr P Richmond, Consultant in Accident and Emergency Medicine, Cardiff Royal Infirmary

Dr G A O Thomas, Consultant Gastroenterologist, University Hospital of Wales

Mr M H Wheeler, Consultant Surgeon, University Hospital of Wales

Professor G T Williams, Consultant Histopathologist, University Hospital of Wales

Mr H Williams, Consultant Ear, Nose and Throat Surgeon, East Glamorgan Hospital

Mr R J L L Williams, Consultant Surgeon, East Glamorgan Hospital

Part I

Questions

General

Case 1

A 40-year-old gentleman presented to the outpatient department with a left-sided groin swelling (Figure 1a).

1.1 What is the diagnosis?

1.2 How common is this condition?

1.3 How should this condition be treated?

1.4 What complications may follow surgery for this condition?

A second patient has a large swelling in his left groin and a suspicion of a swelling on the right. A radiological investigation was performed (Figure 1b).

1.5 What is this investigation and what does it show?

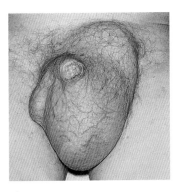

Figure 1a

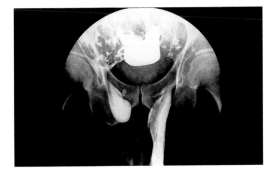

Figure 1b

Case 2

A 40-year-old builder presented with a painless left-sided groin swelling which increased in size on coughing (Figure 2).

2.1 What is the differential diagnosis for this gentleman and what is the likely diagnosis?

2.2 What factors commonly predispose to this condition?

2.3 What is the underlying defect?

2.4 What are the important anatomical relationships?

2.5 How should this gentleman be treated?

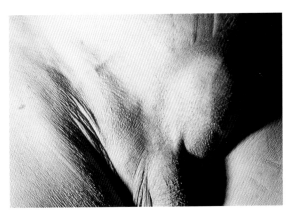

Figure 2

Case 3

A 45-year-old lady housewife attended the clinic with a small lump in her right groin (Figure 3a).

3.1 What is the likely diagnosis?

3.2 What is the aetiology?

3.3 What operative approaches are available?

3.4 What are the complications specific to surgery for this condition?

A second patient was admitted as an emergency with a tender groin swelling and a distended abdomen. An abdominal radiograph was performed (Figure 3b).

3.5 What is the diagnosis?

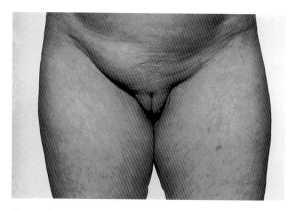

Figure 3a

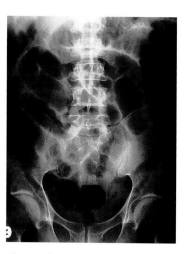

Figure 3b

Case 4

A 50-year-old lady presented with a painless swelling on her anterior abdominal wall (Figure 4).

4.1 What is the likely diagnosis?

4.2 Which patients classically develop this condition?

4.3 Of what is the swelling usually composed?

4.4 What is the pathogenesis of this condition?

4.5 Do all such swellings require surgical treatment?

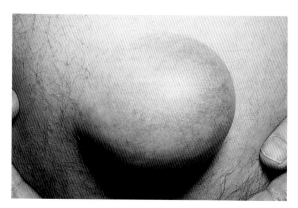

Figure 4

Case 5

A 55-year-old gentleman developed a large swelling in his upper abdomen 2 years after a laparotomy (Figure 5a).

5.1 What is the likely diagnosis?

5.2 What are the important aetiological factors?

5.3 Can any measures be taken to prevent this complication?

5.4 How should this be treated?

A second patient presented with a tender mass in the scar from a previous laparotomy and underwent an emergency operation (Figure 5b).

5.5 What is the diagnosis?

Case 6

A 60-year-old lady who had previously undergone an abdominoperineal resection for a colonic neoplasm presented with a massive swelling of the abdominal wall (Figure 6a).

6.1 What is the diagnosis?

6.2 How common is this complication?

6.3 What symptoms result from this condition?

6.4 How is this condition treated?

A second patient presented with a different complication of surgery (Figure 6b).

6.5 What is the diagnosis?

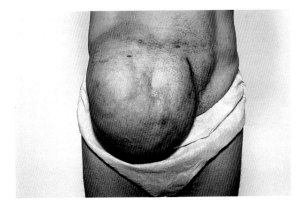

Figure 5a

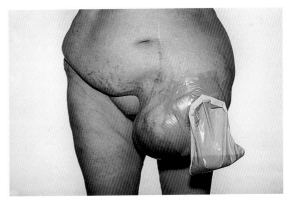

Figure 6a

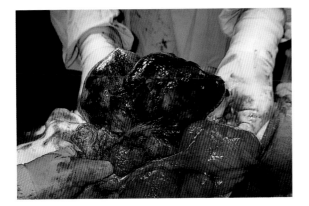

Figure 5b

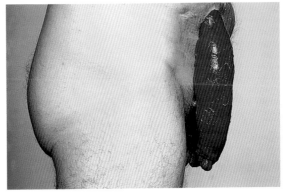

Figure 6b

Case 7

A 20-year-old gentleman presented to the outpatient department with a soft interscapular mass (Figure 7a).

7.1 What is the likely diagnosis?

7.2 What is the pathology of this condition and is there a risk of malignant transformation?

7.3 What are the common anatomical locations for these lesions?

An operation was performed (Figure 7b).

7.4 What characteristics of this lesion are evident?

A second patient presented with multiple swellings of a similar nature (Figure 7c).

7.5 By what eponym is this condition known?

Case 8

An elderly woman presented with a slow growing lesion on the dorsum of her right hand (Figure 8a).

8.1 What features are evident and what is the diagnosis?

8.2 What are the important aetiological factors?

8.3 What treatment options are available?

8.4 What is the prognosis for this condition?

A 40-year-old gentleman who had sustained a full-thickness burn as a child presented with a similar lesion (Figure 8b).

8.5 By what eponym is this lesion known?

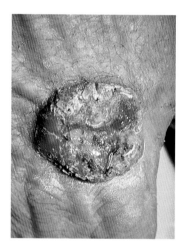

Figure 8a

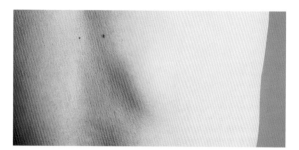

Figure 7a

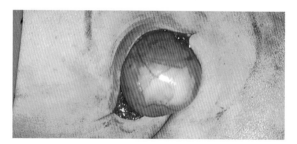

Figure 7b

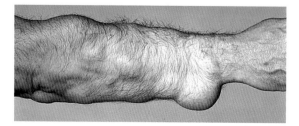

Figure 7c

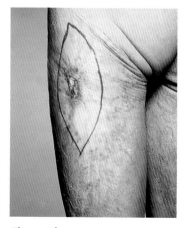

Figure 8b

Case 9

An elderly lady presented with a lesion above her left eye (Figure 9a).

9.1 What features are evident and what is the diagnosis?

9.2 What are the important aetiological factors?

9.3 What is the classical anatomical distribution?

9.4 What are the treatment options and what is the prognosis?

A second patient presented with a similar lesion on her right cheek (Figure 9b).

9.5 What is the diagnosis and what is the important differential diagnosis?

Case 10

A fair-skinned individual was noted to have a pigmented lesion on his back during a routine examination (Figure 10a).

10.1 What is the likely diagnosis and what important features characterise this lesion?

10.2 How is such a lesion treated?

10.3 What are the important prognostic indicators?

A patient who had undergone surgical treatment for a similar lesion on the leg is shown in Figure 10b.

10.4 What is seen and what treatment options are available?

A similar lesion is seen on the face of this woman (Figure 10c).

10.5 What is the diagnosis and how does the prognosis of this lesion compare with the patient shown in Figure 10a?

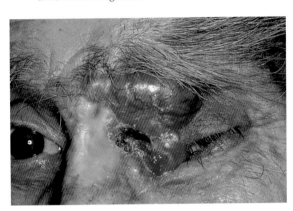

Figure 9a

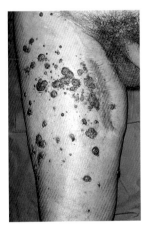

Figure 10a

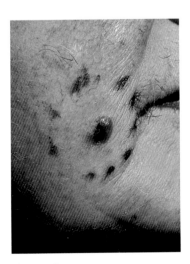

Figure 9b

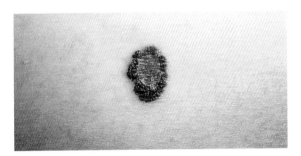

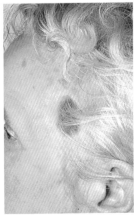

Figure 10b   **Figure 10c**

Case 11

A 50-year-old woman presented with a pigmented lesion under the nail of her left big toe (Figure 11).

11.1 What is the differential diagnosis?

11.2 How should the diagnosis be confirmed?

11.3 Where other than skin may these lesions occur?

11.4 What other regions should be examined?

11.5 What primary treatment should this patient receive?

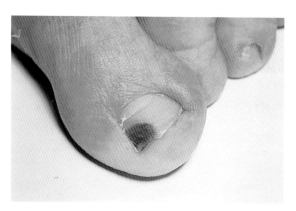

Figure 11

Case 12

A 70-year-old woman presented to the outpatient clinic with a rapidly growing lesion on her right cheek (Figure 12).

12.1 What classical features are seen?

12.2 What is the diagnosis and who is affected by this condition?

12.3 What important differential must be considered?

12.4 How is such a lesion treated?

12.5 Do these lesions recur?

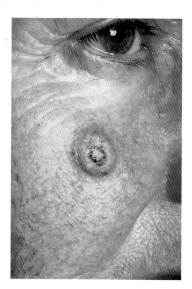

Figure 12

Case 13

A young man attended the outpatient department with a painful left big toe (Figure 13a).

13.1 What is seen and what is the diagnosis?

13.2 Which age group usually suffers from this condition and what is its aetiology?

13.3 What operation should be performed and what are the important principles?

A 50-year-old woman presented to her general practitioner with a different condition affecting her right big toe (Figure 13b).

13.4 What is the diagnosis and what is the underlying pathology?

13.5 How is this condition treated?

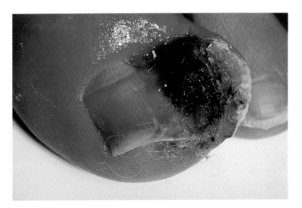

Figure 13a

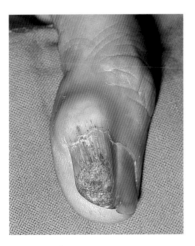

Figure 13b

Case 14

A young man presented to the outpatient department with a soft swelling on his scalp just above the hairline (Figure 14a).

14.1 What is the diagnosis and what is the pathogenesis of this condition?

14.2 Where else may these lesions occur?

14.3 What are their physical characteristics?

14.4 How is such a lesion managed?

A complication of this condition is seen in Figure 14b.

14.5 What is seen and what other complications may occur?

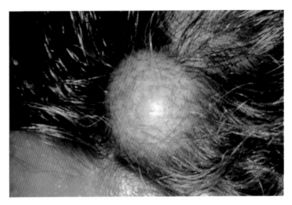

Figure 14a

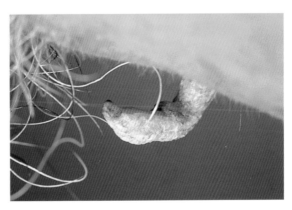

Figure 14b

Case 15

A 50-year-old gentleman presented with a swelling on the dorsum of his left wrist (Figure 15).

15.1 What is the diagnosis?

15.2 What is the typical mode of presentation?

15.3 Where else are these lesions seen?

15.4 What is the proposed aetiology?

15.5 How is such a lesion treated?

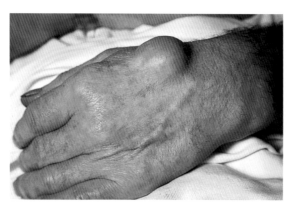

Figure 15

Case 16

A middle-aged gentleman presented with a history of chronic perineal discharge (Figures 16a and 16b).

16.1 What is the diagnosis?

16.2 What is the proposed aetiology of this condition?

16.3 What other regions does the condition commonly affect?

16.4 What treatment options are available?

16.5 What are the results of surgery?

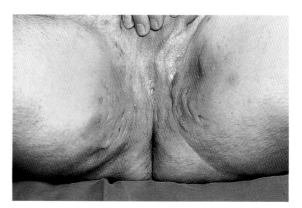

Figure 16a

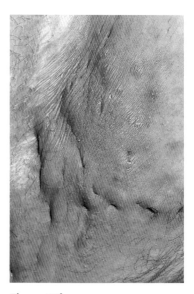

Figure 16b

Case 17

An 8-year-old boy attended the outpatient department with a short history of a bright red lesion on his arm (Figure 17).

17.1 What features are evident?

17.2 What is the diagnosis?

17.3 What is the demography of this condition?

17.4 Is this name appropriate?

17.5 How should this lesion be managed?

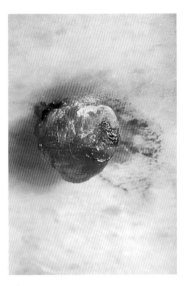

Figure 17

Case 18

A middle-aged woman presented to the surgical outpatients with multiple fleshy skin lesions (Figure 18).

18.1 What is the diagnosis and what other skin lesions may be seen in this condition?

18.2 What are the other modes of presentation?

18.3 What are the important associations of the condition?

18.4 What is the genetic basis of this disease?

18.5 Is any surgical treatment required?

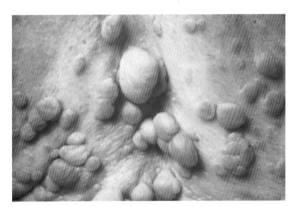

Figure 18

Case 19

An elderly patient on anticoagulant medication for a prosthetic heart valve was admitted as an emergency with a tender right iliac fossa mass.

19.1   What is the differential diagnosis?

On examination the mass was found to be restricted to the anterior abdominal wall. Computerised tomography (CT) was performed to confirm the diagnosis (Figure 19).

19.2   What is seen?

19.3   What are the common aetiological factors?

19.4   What is the pathophysiology of this condition?

19.5   How should this condition be treated?

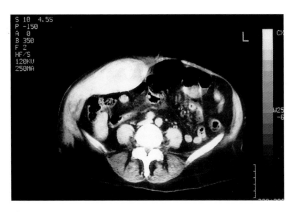

Figure 19

Case 20

An obese diabetic suffered a complication following an emergency laparotomy for perforated diverticular disease (Figure 20).

20.1   What is the diagnosis?

20.2   What are the recognised aetiological factors?

20.3   Which organisms are commonly isolated?

20.4   How should this patient be treated?

20.5   What further complication may ensue if this patient is left untreated?

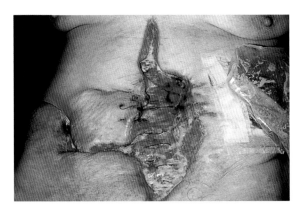

Figure 20

Upper gastrointestinal

Case 21

The patient is a 62-year-old male, non-smoker who has suffered with heartburn and acid regurgitation for a number of years. Over the last 2 months he has developed dysphagia to solids. General examination is unremarkable. Respiratory function tests and echocardiography are normal.

21.1 What investigations are shown (Figures 21a and 21b) and what do they demonstrate?

21.2 What is the TNM classification of this disease?

21.3 What operations may be performed for this disease?

21.4 What are the complications of surgery?

21.5 What is the post-operative mortality of surgery for this condition? What is the likelihood that this gentleman will survive 5 years?

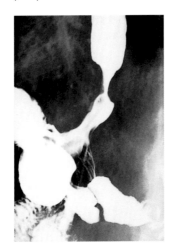

Figure 21a

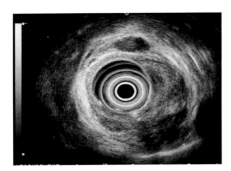

Figure 21b

Case 22

The patient is a 70-year-old male, lifelong smoker who has developed dysphagia to solids over the last 3 months. In addition, he has noticed a lump in the left supraclavicular fossa. Respiratory function reveals an FEV1 of 0.8 L/min.

22.1 What investigations are shown (Figures 22a and 22b) and what do they demonstrate?

22.2 What is the epidemiology of this condition?

22.3 Discuss the factors that would influence the treatment of this gentleman.

22.4 What would be appropriate treatment(s)?

22.5 What are the risk factors for this condition?

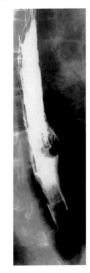

Figure 22a

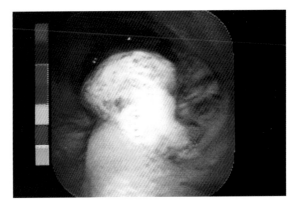

Figure 22b

Case 23

These endoscopic photographs (Figures 23a and 23b) were obtained from two patients with symptoms of heartburn and acid regurgitation.

23.1 What do they show?

23.2 What is the usual method of grading this disease?

23.3 What is the usual means of treatment? What is the sinister complication of the condition shown in Figure 23b?

23.4 If the disease is refractory to the above therapy what would be the next investigation of choice?

23.5 What would the appropriate treatment be for symptoms refractory to the initial therapy?

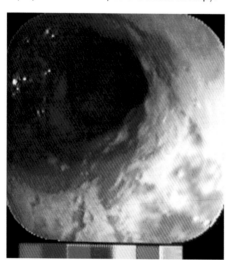

Figure 23a

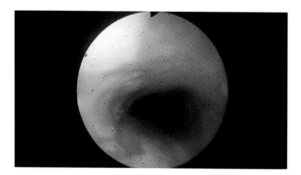

Figure 23b

Case 24

The patient is a 30-year-old female with a 24 month history of dysphagia, weight loss and food regurgitation.

24.1 What investigations are shown (Figures 24a–c) and what abnormalities are shown in Figure 24a?

24.2 What are the characteristic findings of the investigation in Figure 24b in this condition?

24.3 What is the epidemiology of this condition?

24.4 Would you expect to find abnormalities at endoscopy in this condition?

24.5 What is the treatment of this condition and what are its complications?

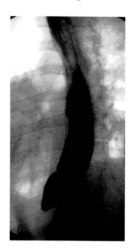

Figure 24a

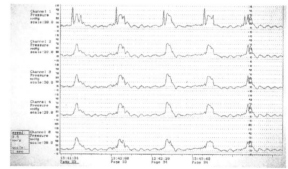

Figure 24b

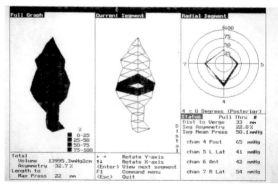

Figure 24c

Case 25

The patient is a 45-year-old male who has been taking indomethacin for 3 years for back pain. He gives a 48 hour history of abdominal pain. Initially the pain was localised to the epigastrium, but latterly it increased in severity and became more generalised.

25.1 What do Figures 25a and 25b show?

25.2 What are the typical presenting features of this condition?

25.3 What is the management of this condition?

25.4 What are the other complications of this condition?

25.5 Who is principally affected by this condition? What are the predisposing factors?

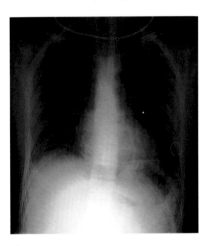

Figure 25a

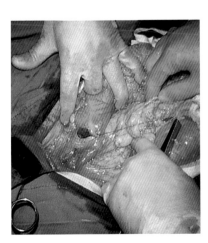

Figure 25b

Case 26

A male aged 65 presents to the rapid access gastroscopy clinic with a 4 month history of epigastric pain and weight loss. He has been treated empirically with an H2-receptor antagonist to no avail. He undergoes gastroscopy and subsequently an operation. The endoscopic findings are shown in Figure 26a and the surgical resection specimen in Figure 26b.

26.1 What is the likely diagnosis?

26.2 What is the epidemiology of this condition?

26.3 What changes have been seen in the incidence of this condition in the UK? With what condition does it show common features epidemiologically?

26.4 What is the aetiology of this condition?

26.5 What is the treatment of this condition?

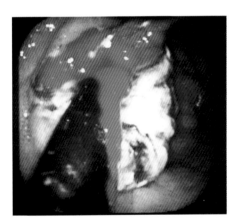

Figure 26a

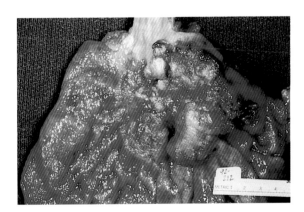

Figure 26b

Case 27

Figures 27a and 27b are from a 45-year-old patient undergoing foregut investigation and treatment. Biopsies have been taken from the lesion on three occasions. The first two sets of biopsies showed normal gastric mucosa only. On the third occasion biopsies showed a spindle cell lesion in the submucosa.

27.1 What is shown in Figures 27a and 27b?

27.2 Based upon the appearances shown in Figure 27a what is the differential diagnosis?

27.3 What is the epidemiology of this condition?

27.4 What are the presenting features of this disease?

27.5 What is the treatment of this condition?

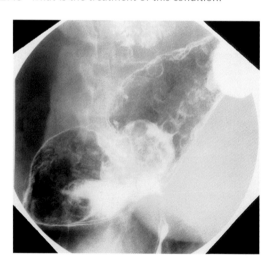

Figure 27a

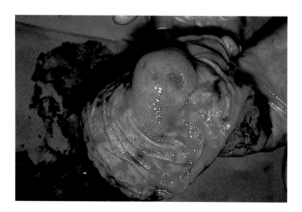

Figure 27b

Case 28

The patient is a 45-year-old male presenting for the first time to the Accident and Emergency Department vomiting fresh blood.

28.1 What is shown in Figures 28a–c? What is the diagnosis?

28.2 What is the underlying pathophysiology of this condition?

28.3 What is the appropriate emergency treatment for this patient?

28.4 What are the complications of treatment?

28.5 How may the underlying pathophysiology be altered in an elective setting?

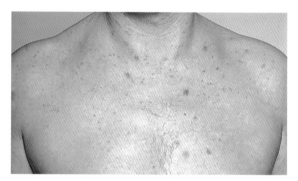

Figure 28a

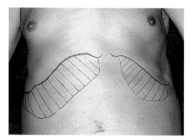

Figure 28b

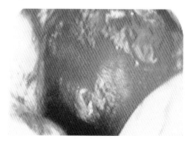

Figure 28c

Case 29

Endoscopic examination (Figure 29) was performed on a 45-year-old male with a 6 month history of epigastric pain.

29.1 What is the diagnosis?

29.2 What infective agent is associated with this condition, and how may its presence be confirmed?

29.3 How is the infective agent treated?

29.4 What follow-up should this patient have?

29.5 Who typically develops this condition and what are the predisposing factors?

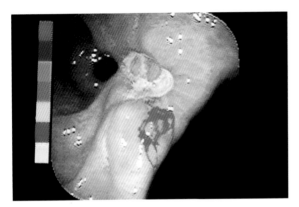

Figure 29

Case 30

Further to the investigation shown (Figure 30), a 76-year-old male patient has undergone gastroscopy and biopsy of the abnormality indicated in the picture on two separate occasions. Both sets of biopsies revealed chronic inflammation only.

30.1 What is the likely diagnosis?

30.2 What is the aetiology of the condition in the patient described?

30.3 What are the other causes of this condition?

30.4 What are the presenting features of this condition?

30.5 What is the treatment of this condition?

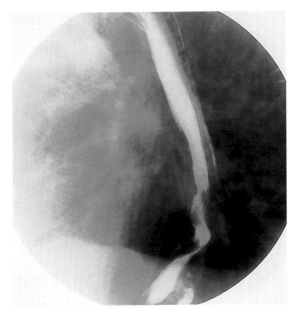

Figure 30

Case 31

Figure 31 depicts a common surgical complication.

31.1 What is shown in Figure 31 and what is the diagnosis?

31.2 What is the aetiology of this condition?

31.3 What is the microbiology of this condition?

31.4 What other findings may Figure 31 show in this condition? What other imaging techniques may be helpful?

31.5 What is the treatment of this condition?

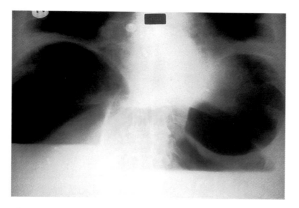

Figure 31

Hepatobiliary and pancreas

Case 32

An 80-year-old lady presented with a history of progressively deepening painless jaundice, pale stools and dark urine.

32.1 What is the differential diagnosis?

An ultrasound scan was performed (Figure 32a).

32.2 What does it show?

A second radiological procedure was performed (Figure 32b).

32.3 What is this procedure and what does it show?

32.4 What is being carried out in Figures 32c and 32d?

32.5 What other options are available and what is the prognosis for this condition?

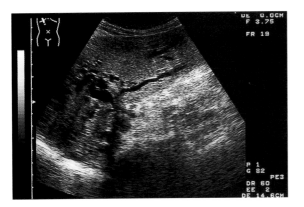

Figure 32a

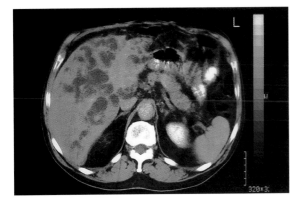

Figure 32b

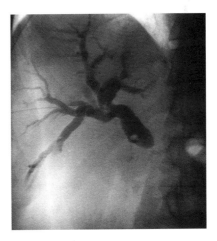

Figure 32c

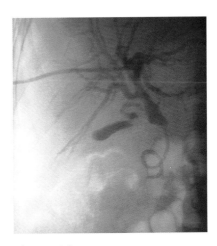

Figure 32d

Case 33

A 48-year-old farmer presented with a history of fever and right upper quadrant discomfort.

33.1 What is the likely diagnosis and what diagnostic serological tests may be performed?

A CT was performed (Figure 33a).

33.2 What does it show and why is it useful?

33.3 What are the management options?

The patient underwent an operation (Figure 33b).

33.4 What are the principles of operating on this condition?

33.5 What are the results of surgery?

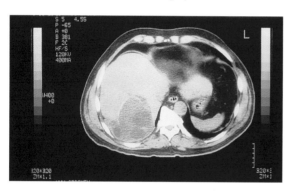

Figure 33a

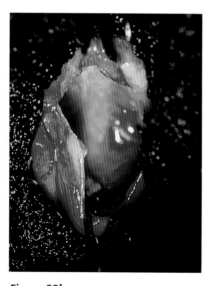

Figure 33b

Case 34

A 60-year-old woman presented with a painful right upper quadrant mass. An ultrasound scan was performed (Figure 34a).

34.1 What is seen in Figure 34a?

A CT was performed.

34.2 What is the diagnosis?

34.3 What are the common pathologies?

35.4 What are the recognised predisposing factors?

34.5 What are the management options and what is the prognosis of this condition?

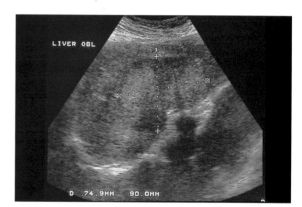

Figure 34a

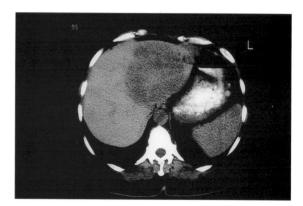

Figure 34b

Case 35

A 40-year-old woman presented as an emergency with upper abdominal pain. A plain abdominal radiograph was performed (Figure 35a).

35.1 What is seen in Figure 35a and what is the likely diagnosis?

35.2 What does the ultrasound shown in Figure 35b demonstrate?

35.3 What is the prevalence of this condition?

35.4 What are the recognised predisposing factors?

35.5 What complication is seen in Figures 35c and 35d and what other complications may occur?

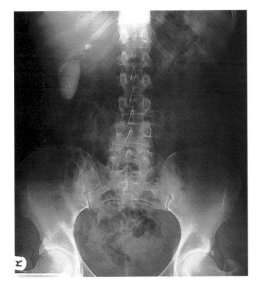

Figure 35a

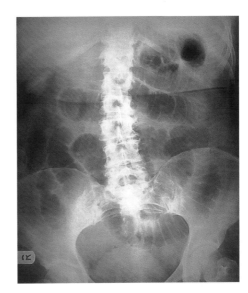

Figure 35c

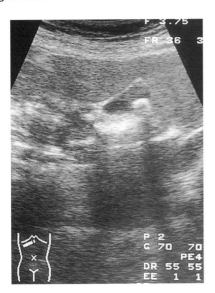

Figure 35b

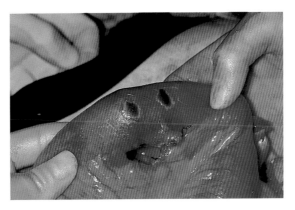

Figure 35d

Case 36

A 44-year-old woman presented with jaundice following a laparoscopic cholecystectomy.

36.1 What is the differential diagnosis?

A radiological procedure was performed (Figures 36a and 36b).

36.2 What is seen?

36.3 What alternative procedures are seen in Figures 36c and 36d?

36.4 What are the recognised complications of this procedure?

36.5 What are the other treatment options?

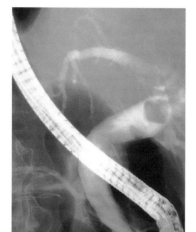

Figure 36a

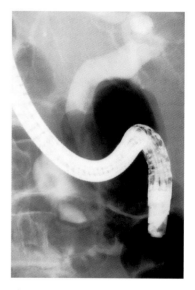

Figure 36c

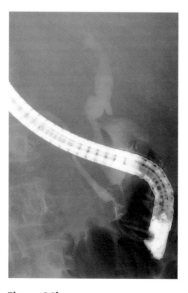

Figure 36b

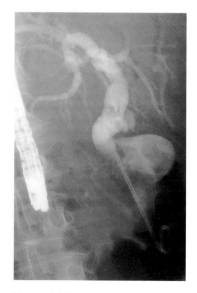

Figure 36d

Case 37

A 49-year-old with a history of gallstones was admitted as an emergency.

A plain abdominal film was taken (Figure 37a).

37.1 What is seen and what is the likely diagnosis?

37.2 What is Charcot's triad?

An ultrasound of the gallbladder was performed (Figure 37b)

37.3 What is seen?

A CT was performed (Figure 37c).

37.4 What does it show?

37.5 How is this complication managed?

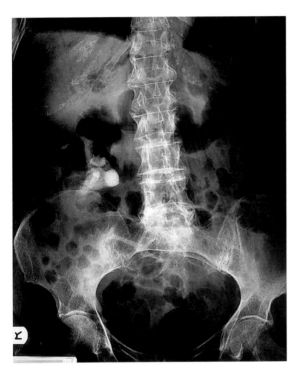

Figure 37a

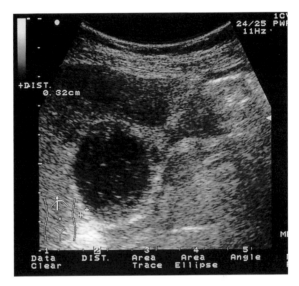

Figure 37b

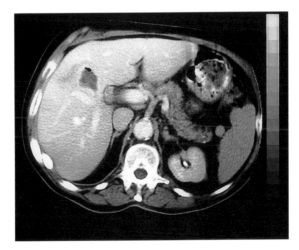

Figure 37c

Case 38

A patient with gallstones was admitted for a routine procedure.

38.1 What procedure is being carried out (Figure 38a) and what are the important safety checks?

38.2 What is being carried out in Figures 38b and 38c?

38.3 What structures define Calot's triangle and what is its importance?

38.4 What is demonstrated in Figure 38d and is this a routine procedure?

38.5 What are the complications of this procedure?

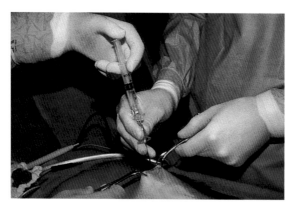

Figure 38a

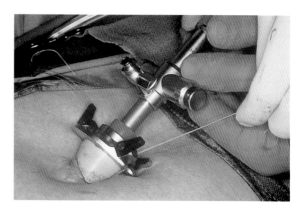

Figure 38c

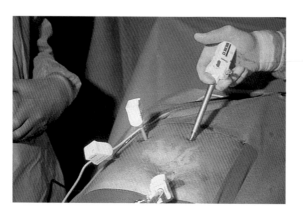

Figure 38b

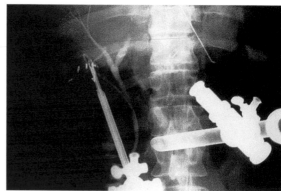

Figure 38d

Case 39

This patient presented was discharged 24 hours after a laparoscopic cholecystectomy and then re-presented after a further 48 hours with progressive jaundice.

39.1 What is the likely diagnosis?

39.2 What investigation is being performed in Figure 39a, and what does it show?

39.3 What are the causative mechanisms?

39.4 What are the treatment options?

A second patient sustained a different complication (Figure 39b).

39.5 What is seen and what is the usual aetiology?

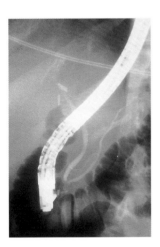

Figure 39a

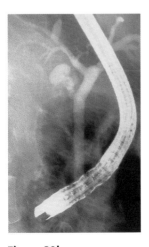

Figure 39b

Case 40

A 40-year-old woman presented as an emergency with epigastric pain and vomiting. Laboratory investigations revealed a serum amylase of 1500 IU/L.

40.1 What clinical sign is seen (Figure 40a), what is the likely diagnosis and what is the differential?

40.2 What are Imrie's criteria?

40.3 What are the common aetiologies of this condition?

A CT scan was performed (Figure 40b).

40.4 What does it show?

40.5 What are the principles of management?

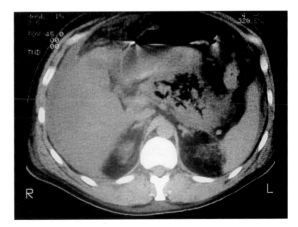

Figure 40a

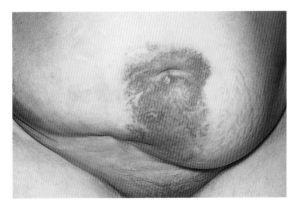

Figure 40b

Case 41

A 32-year-old who was recovering from an episode of acute pancreatitis attended the outpatient department with an epigastric mass. A CT was performed (Figure 41a).

41.1 What is seen in Figure 41a?

41.2 What is the aetiology of this condition?

41.3 An interventional radiological procedure was performed (Figure 41b). What was done?

41.4 What other treatment options are available?

41.5 What are the main complications of acute pancreatitis?

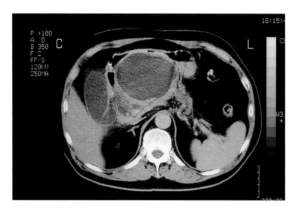

Figure 41a

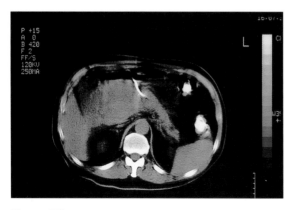

Figure 41b

Case 42

A 45-year-old alcoholic presented with severe upper abdominal pain.

An endoscopic investigation was performed to assess the condition.

42.1 What is seen in Figure 42?

42.2 What are the recognised aetiological factors?

42.3 What medical treatment options are available?

42.4 What operations may be used to treat this condition?

42.5 What are the results of surgery?

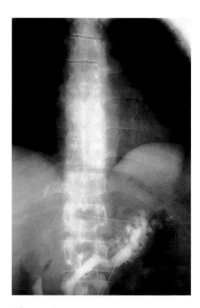

Figure 42

Case 43

A 73-year-old woman presented with painless jaundice and a mass in the right upper quadrant.

43.1 What does Courvoisier's Law state?

An endoscopic diagnostic procedure was performed (Figure 43a).

43.2 What is seen and why is this test useful?

A CT was performed (Figure 43b).

43.3 What is seen and why was it performed?

43.4 What are the important aetiological factors?

43.5 How should this condition be treated and what is the outlook?

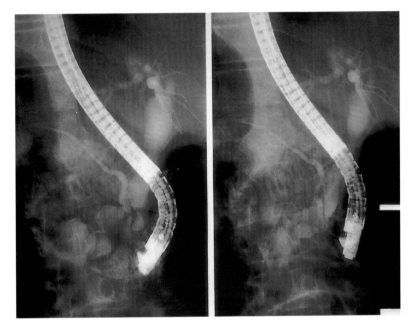

Figure 43a

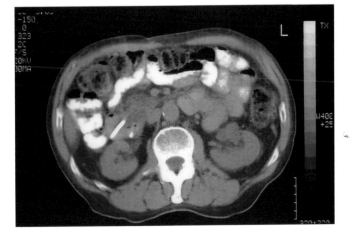

Figure 43b

Case 44

A 64-year-old woman was investigated for vague right upper quadrant pain.

An ultrasound scan was performed (Figure 44a).

44.1 What is seen?

44.2 How should this condition be treated?

44.3 What is the prognosis?

After an initially successful operation, she re-presented after 18 months with obstructive jaundice. A radiological investigation was performed.

44.4 What is shown in Figure 44b and Figure 44c?

44.5 If this condition was identified at the time of laparoscopic cholecystectomy, what would the treatment be?

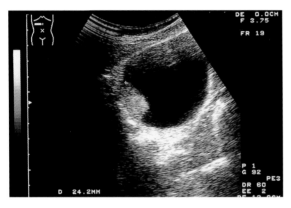

Figure 44a

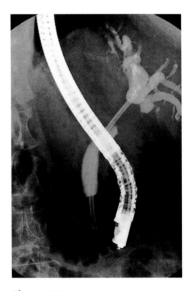

Figure 44c

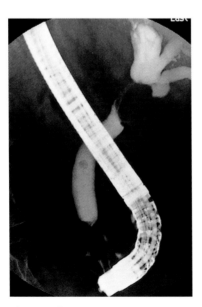

Figure 44b

Lower gastrointestinal

Case 45

Figures 45a–d relate to several patients with the same condition.

45.1 What do Figures 45a–c show and what is the diagnosis?

45.2 What is the epidemiology of this condition and what condition does it share epidemiological similarities with?

45.3 What is shown in Figure 45d? Is it always found?

45.4 What are the complications of the disease?

45.5 What proportion of patients will ultimately require surgery? What are the two commonly employed operations for disease affecting the small bowel?

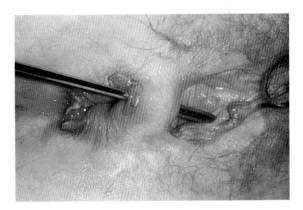

Figure 45c

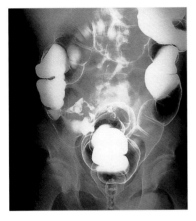

Figure 45a

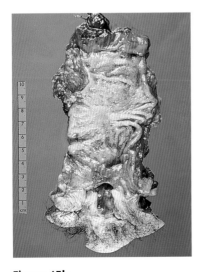

Figure 45b

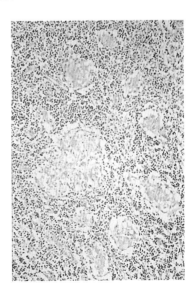

Figure 45d

Case 46

The patient is a 30-year-old male with a 4 week history of diarrhoea, rectal bleeding, abdominal pain and weight loss. Over the last 24 hours the abdominal pain has increased in severity, and the frequency of bowel action has increased. Examination reveals fever and tachycardia. A plain abdominal radiograph (Figure 46a) was performed. Figure 46b was taken at the time of surgery.

46.1 What is the most likely diagnosis?

46.2 Is this the usual mode of presentation for this condition? What other conditions may present in this way?

46.3 What are the extra-intestinal manifestations of this condition?

46.4 What are the complications of this disease?

46.5 What is the medical and surgical management of this condition?

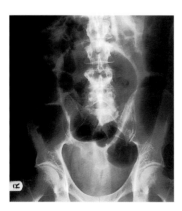

Figure 46a

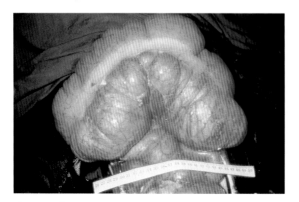

Figure 46b

Case 47

Figure 47a is the per-operative photograph from a 14-year-old boy who presented with a 48 hour history of abdominal pain. Initially the pain was poorly localised to the periumbilical region, but latterly it increased in severity and become localised to the right iliac fossa. Figure 47b is the per-operative photograph from another patient with the same condition.

47.1 What is the diagnosis of the patients seen in Figures 47a and 47b? What features in the history of the patient seen in Figure 47a support this?

47.2 In which patient groups is the morbidity and mortality from this condition greater?

47.3 How does the procedure depicted in Figure 47b differ from that in Figure 47a? What age and sex is the patient shown in Figure 47b most likely to be? Justify your answer.

47.4 Give the names of two individuals whose names are associated with this condition. For both give the feature for which they are remembered.

47.5 What malignant neoplasms most commonly affect this organ?

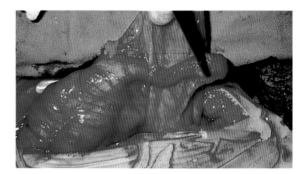

Figure 47a

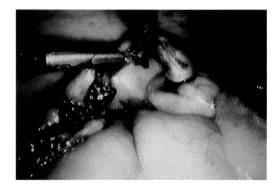

Figure 47b

Case 48

Figure 48a shows the findings at surgery for a congenital condition.

48.1 What is the diagnosis? What embryologic remnant does it represent?

48.2 What investigation is shown in Figure 48b? Is it abnormal in every case?

48.3 How common is this condition? Is it always symptomatic?

48.4 What are the complications of this condition?

48.5 What is the treatment of this condition?

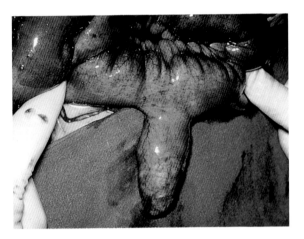

Figure 48a

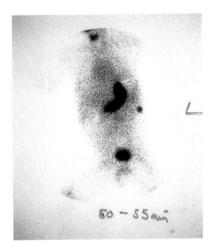

Figure 48b

Case 49

The patient is a 65-year-old male with a 48 hour history of left iliac fossa pain. Examination reveals a fever and localised tenderness. A complication of this condition is shown in Figures 49c and 49d.

49.1 What is shown by Figures 49a and 49b? What is the diagnosis?

49.2 What are the histopathological features of this condition? What is the usual distribution of this condition in the organ that it affects?

49.3 What imaging techniques have been used in Figures 49c and 49d and what is the complication? What are the other complications of this condition?

49.4 Why is the name of this condition a misnomer?

49.5 What is the epidemiology of this condition?

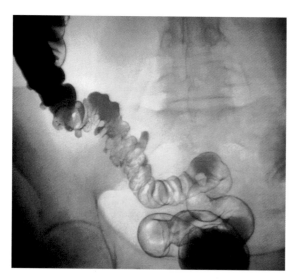

Figure 49a

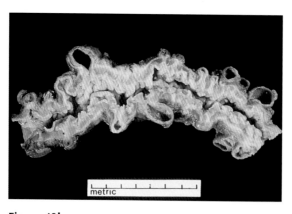

Figure 49b

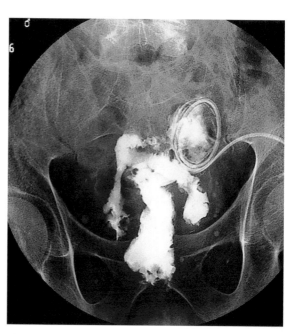

Figure 49c

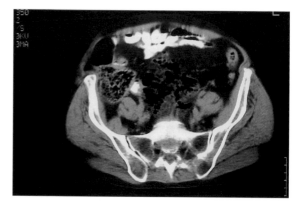

Figure 49d

Case 50

The patient is a 42-year-old female admitted as an emergency with a 24 hour history of progressive abdominal distension, abdominal pain, nausea and vomiting. Figures 50a and 50b were obtained at admission. Over the first 24 hours following hospitalisation the patient's clinical condition deteriorated and she underwent laparotomy. The findings are indicated in Figure 50c.

50.1 What investigations are shown (Figures 50a, 50b) and what features do they indicate?

50.2 What does the per-operative image (Figure 50c) show?

50.3 What are the usual causes of this condition?

50.4 What is the management of this condition?

50.5 What investigation may be used to confirm the diagnosis?

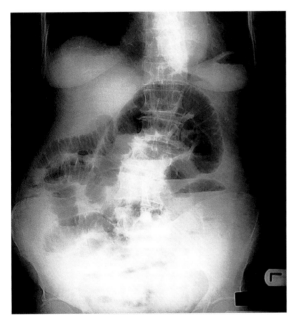

Figure 50a

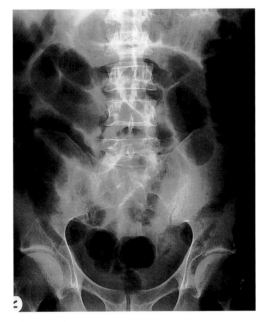

Figure 50b

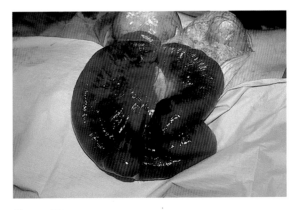

Figure 50c

Case 51

A 69-year-old male is noted to be suffering from iron-deficiency anaemia by his general practitioner. Systemic enquiry is unremarkable.

51.1 What are the initial investigations of iron-deficiency anaemia?

51.2 What investigation is shown (Figure 51a); what is the abnormality affecting the transverse colon, and the likely diagnosis?

51.3 What is the treatment of this disease?

51.4 How might histopathology be useful in predicting the prognosis of the patient? Expand on your answer.

51.5 What complication is shown in Figure 51b?

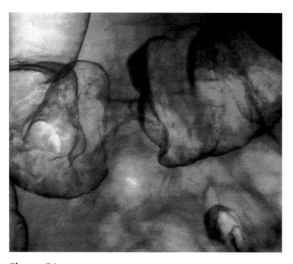

Figure 51a

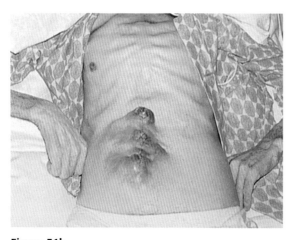

Figure 51b

Case 52

The patient is a 36-year-old male who is admitted with a 24 hour history of acute perianal pain (Figure 52).

52.1 What is the diagnosis?

52.2 What is the other main complication of this condition?

52.3 What is the treatment of this condition in this case and in the outpatient setting?

52.4 What anatomic landmark is it important to be aware of when treating this condition as an outpatient procedure?

52.5 What agent is prescribed following surgical treatment of this condition?

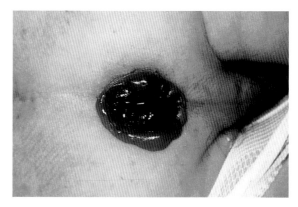

Figure 52

Case 53

Figures 53a and 53b are from a 56-year-old male with a 72 hour history of progressive abdominal distension and colicky-type lower abdominal pain. He had not opened his bowels for 4 days. Further questioning reveals that over the last 4 months he had become constipated. Figures 53c and 53d relate to another patient with the same condition.

53.1 What is shown in Figures 53a and 53b?

53.2 What is the appropriate surgery for this patient and what is the treatment of this condition in the elective setting?

53.3 What investigations are shown in Figures 53c and 53d? What are the findings?

53.4 What are the indications for resectional surgery for disease at this site?

53.5 What chemotherapeutic agent has been most extensively used to treat this disease? How is it administered and what are its adverse effects?

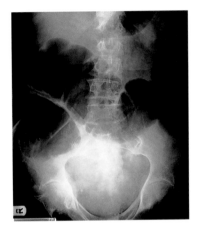

Figure 53a

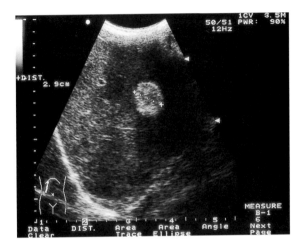

Figure 53c

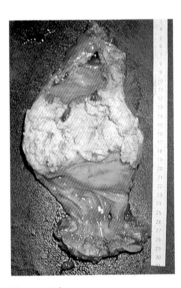

Figure 53b

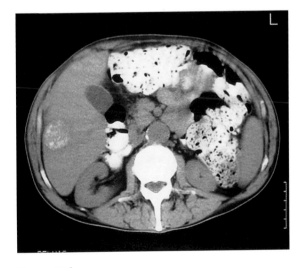

Figure 53d

Case 54

A 15-year-old boy undergoes surgery for an inherited condition (Figure 54).

54.1 What is the diagnosis?

54.2 What is the genetic basis for the condition?

54.3 What associated features may be seen as part of this condition?

54.4 What is the surgical management strategy for this condition?

54.5 Following successful surgery what is the main cause of subsequent mortality in these patients?

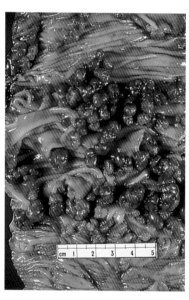

Figure 54

Case 55

A 76-year-old male with Parkinson's disease develops abdominal pain and distension.

55.1 What is shown in Figures 55a and 55b, and what is the diagnosis?

55.2 What is the anatomic prerequisite for an organ to be affected by this condition? Define the condition.

55.3 Is this the most commonly affected site? Which other areas may be affected?

55.4 What is the epidemiology of this condition?

55.5 What is the treatment of this condition?

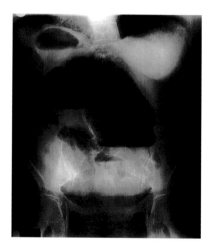

Figure 55a

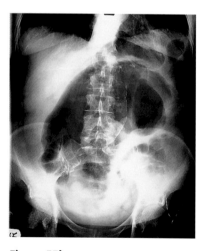

Figure 55b

Case 56

Figures 56a and 56b show a common perianal problem.

56.1 What is shown in the two pictures?

56.2 What features suggest the presence of a fistula-in-ano?

56.3 Who commonly develops this condition?

56.4 What is the management of this condition?

56.5 What is Goodsall's rule?

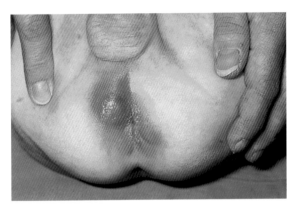

Figure 56a

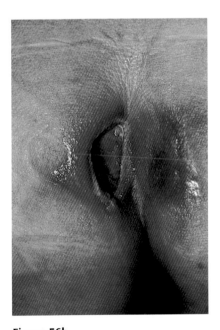

Figure 56b

Case 57

An elderly male patient has experienced left iliac fossa pain intermittently for several months. He underwent an examination (Figure 57).

57.1 What abnormality is shown?

57.2 What are the presenting features of this condition?

57.3 What are the causes of this condition? Which three causes account for around 90% of cases in the UK?

57.4 Is there any difference in the occurrence of this condition between males and females? Justify your answer.

57.5 What is the treatment of this condition?

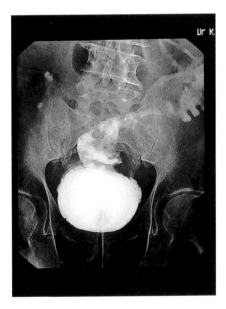

Figure 57

Case 58

The picture shows the findings at laparotomy in an elderly patient with signs of peritonitis (Figure 58).

58.1 What is the diagnosis?

58.2 What are the causes of this condition?

58.3 What are the clinical features of this illness?

58.4 Of the layers that make up the intestinal wall which is affected by this disease process initially?

58.5 What is the treatment of this condition?

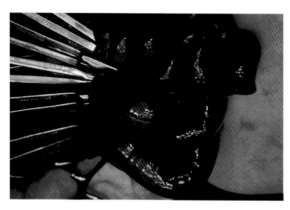

Figure 58

Case 59

A patient with a condition (Figure 59a) has undergone an operation. The per-operative (Figure 59b) and immediate post-operative (Figure 59c) appearances are shown.

59.1 What is the diagnosis (Figure 59a) and what operation is shown (Figures 59b, 59c)?

59.2 Who is affected by this condition?

59.3 What are the predisposing factors?

59.4 What symptom is common in patients with this problem?

59.5 How is the condition managed?

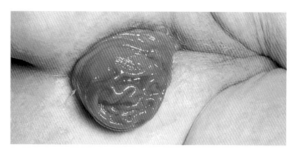

Figure 59a

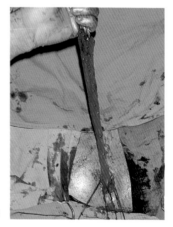

Figure 59b

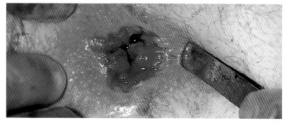

Figure 59c

Case 60

Figure 60 is from a patient presenting to the outpatient clinic with perianal pain.

60.1 What is the diagnosis?

60.2 Who is affected?

60.3 What is the treatment of this condition in the acute and chronic settings?

60.4 What are the main complications of operative treatment?

60.5 Which is the preferred surgical option? What are the advantages and disadvantages of each of the methods of operative treatment?

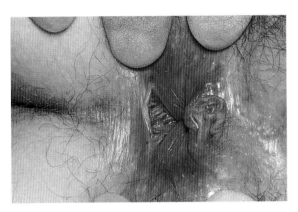

Figure 60

Case 61

Figures 61a–c relate to the insertion of two different feeding devices.

61.1 What is being placed in Figure 61a?

61.2 Which group of patients may benefit from its insertion?

61.3 What is being placed in Figures 61b and 61c?

61.4 Which group of patients are likely to benefit from it?

61.5 What are the complications of the devices shown?

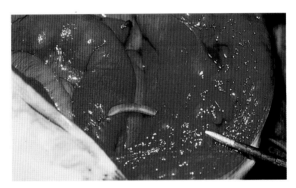

Figure 61a

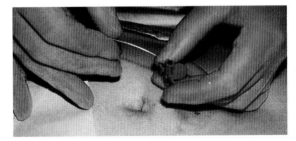

Figure 61b

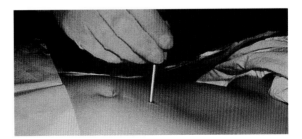

Figure 61c

Case 62

The patient, a male smoker aged 57 years, has received treatment for a neoplasm 6 years earlier. The patient has undergone a laparotomy (findings shown in Figure 62) for a complication relating to the earlier treatment.

62.1 What previous treatment has this patient received and what is the diagnosis? What factors increase the chance of this occurring?

62.2 What diseases is this treatment commonly used for?

62.3 What is the pathogenesis of this complication?

62.4 What are the immediate effects of this treatment on the intestine and how may they be treated?

62.5 How is the complication above diagnosed and treated?

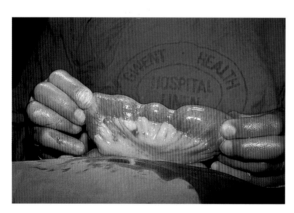

Figure 62

Case 63

The patient indicated in Figure 63 is seen in the outpatient clinic with a perianal problem.

63.1 What is the diagnosis?

63.2 How are such lesions typically classified?

63.3 What is the aetiology of this condition?

63.4 What are the presenting features of this condition?

63.5 What is the treatment of this condition?

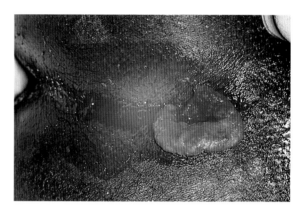

Figure 63

Breast

Case 64

A 30-year-old woman presented as an emergency with a painful right breast (Figure 64a).

64.1 What features are evident?

64.2 What is the likely diagnosis and what important differential diagnosis must be excluded?

64.3 What group is classically said to suffer from this condition?

64.4 Which organisms are usually isolated?

An operation was performed (Figure 64b).

64.5 What are the important principles of surgery for this condition?

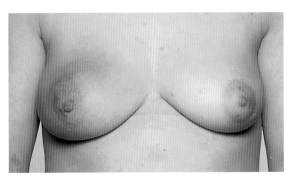

Figure 64a

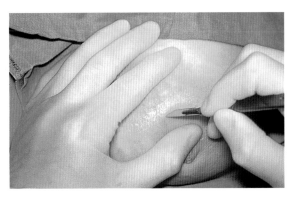

Figure 64b

Case 65

A 19-year-old girl presented with a discrete mass in the upper inner quadrant of the right breast.

A radiological examination was performed (Figure 65).

65.1 What is this investigation and what does it show?

65.2 What are the characteristic clinical features of this type of lesion?

65.3 What are the demographic characteristics of this condition?

65.4 Is this condition associated with a risk of malignancy?

65.5 What treatment options are available?

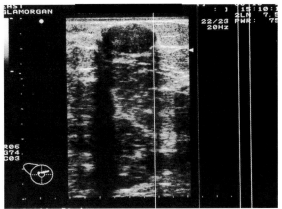

Figure 65

Case 66

A 40-year-old woman presented to the outpatient department with multiple lumps in both breasts. A mammogram was performed (Figure 66a).

66.1 What is evident on the mammograms and what is the likely diagnosis?

66.2 What is the usual mode of presentation?

66.3 What is the aetiology of this condition?

66.4 What procedure is being carried out in Figure 66b?

66.5 What other treatment is required?

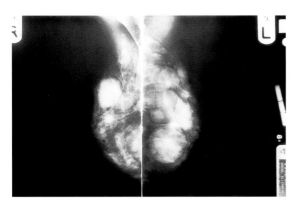

Figure 66a

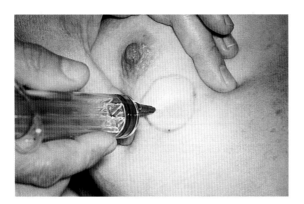

Figure 66b

Case 67

A 50-year-old lady presented with an itchy, erythematous lesion affecting her left breast.

67.1 What is seen?

67.2 What is the diagnosis?

67.3 What is the histology of this condition?

67.4 Where else is this condition seen?

67.5 How should such a case be treated?

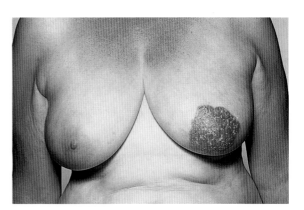

Figure 67

Case 68

A 35-year-old lady presented to the breast clinic with a bloody discharge from her right nipple (Figure 68a).

68.1 What is the differential diagnosis?

68.2 What is the treatment for the most common cause of this symptom?

68.3 A second woman presented with a toothpaste-like discharge (Figure 68b). What is the likely diagnosis?

68.4 What is the aetiology of this condition?

68.5 What are the treatment options available?

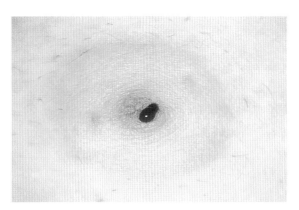

Figure 68a

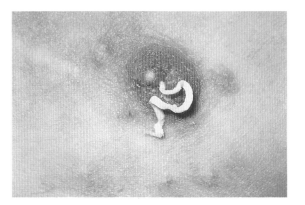

Figure 68b

Case 69

A middle-aged male presented with tender symmetrical enlargement of his breasts (Figure 69).

69.1 What is the diagnosis?

69.2 What is the pathogenesis?

69.3 What are the common aetiological factors?

69.4 How is the diagnosis confirmed?

69.5 How is the condition treated?

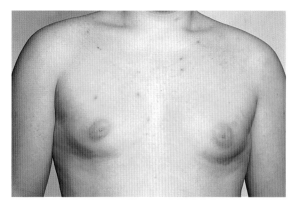

Figure 69

Case 70

A 58-year-old woman was called to her local breast unit following a screening mammogram. A repeat mammogram was performed (Figure 70a).

70.1 What does the mammogram show?

70.2 How common is this condition?

70.3 What is illustrated in Figure 70b?

70.4 What further treatment is required?

70.5 What is the prognosis for this condition?

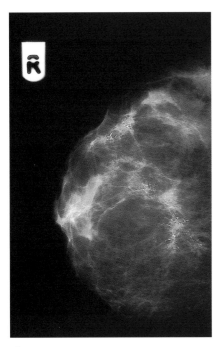

Figure 70a

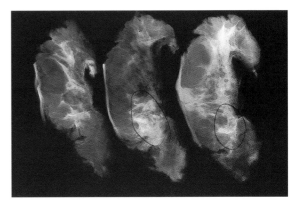

Figure 70b

Case 71

A 60-year-old woman attended her breast unit following a screening mammogram (Figures 71a and 71b). Clinical examination was normal.

71.1 What views are illustrated and what do they show?

71.2 A second radiological diagnostic procedure was performed. What is seen in Figure 71c?

71.3 How may a cytological diagnosis be obtained?

71.4 How is breast cytology classified?

A second patient with a similar lesion underwent an operation.

71.5 What is shown in Figure 71d?

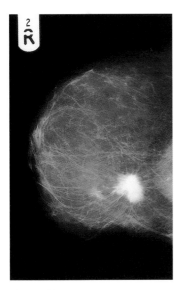

Figure 71a

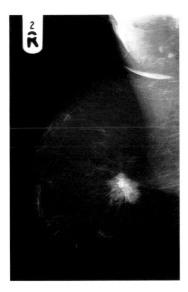

Figure 71b

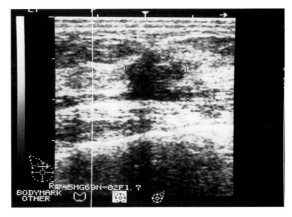

Figure 71c

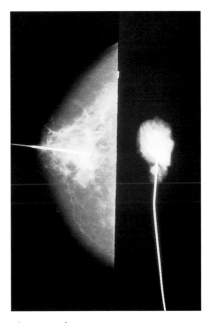

Figure 71d

Case 72

A 65-year-old woman presented to the breast clinic having noted a small lump in her right breast whilst showering.

Mammography was performed (Figures 72a and 72b).

72.1 What is seen and what is the diagnosis?

72.2 How common is this condition?

72.3 What are the important aetiological factors?

72.4 How is this condition classified and give the classification?

72.5 What treatment options would be appropriate for this lady and what is her prognosis?

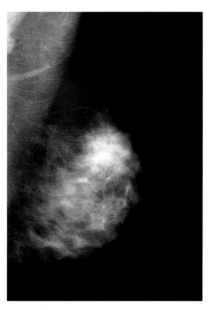

Figure 72a

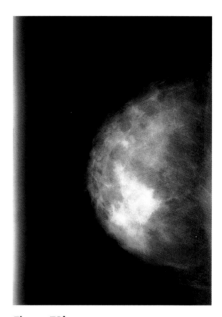

Figure 72b

Case 73

A 70-year-old widow presented with a lesion in the left breast (Figure 73).

73.1 What features are seen?

73.2 What is the likely diagnosis?

73.3 What other regions need to be examined?

73.4 How is such a lesion treated?

73.5 What is the prognosis for such a case?

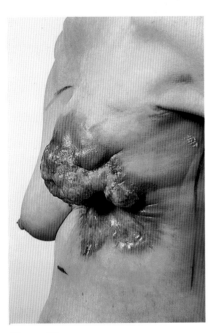

Figure 73

Case 74

A 60-year-old lady who had previously undergone a left mastectomy presented to the outpatient department with a firm nodule in her scar (Figure 74a).

74.1 What is the likely diagnosis?

74.2 How is the diagnosis confirmed?

She also noted a recent history of chest pain and shortness of breath and a chest radiograph was performed (Figure 74b).

74.3 What is seen?

74.4 What other problems are associated with this disease process?

74.5 What management options are available?

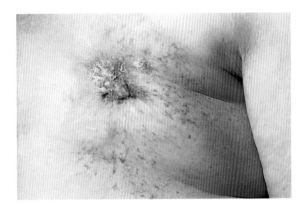

Figure 74a

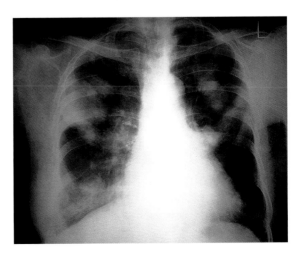

Figure 74b

Case 75

A 57-year-old woman with a rapidly growing mass in her left breast (Figure 75).

75.1 What is seen?

75.2 What is the likely diagnosis?

75.3 What investigations should be performed?

75.4 Do such masses have malignant potential?

75.5 What is the recommended treatment for such a lesion?

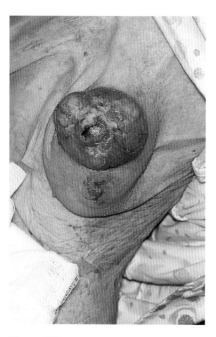

Figure 75

Endocrine

Case 76

A 50-year-old gentleman presented with this characteristic facial flushing (Figure 76a).

76.1 What is the likely diagnosis?

76.2 How else may this condition present?

76.3 How is the diagnosis confirmed?

An operation was performed (Figures 76b and 76c)

76.4 What is the pathophysiology of this condition?

76.5 What are the operative findings and what treatment options are available?

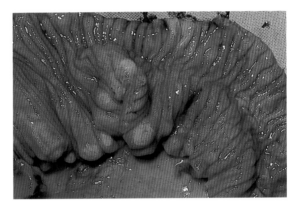

Figure 76b

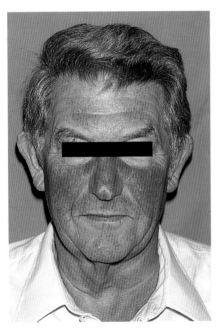

Figure 76a

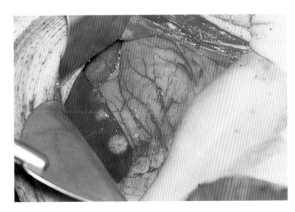

Figure 76c

Case 77

A 45-year-old lady presented to the ophthalmology clinic before being referred to a surgeon (Figure 77a).

77.1 What features are evident and what is the diagnosis?

77.2 What are the typical biochemical features of this disease?

Examination of her legs revealed characteristic features (Figure 77b).

77.3 What is seen?

77.4 What pre-operative investigations are required?

77.5 What treatment options are available?

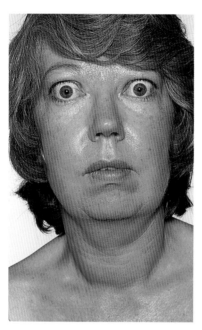

Figure 77a

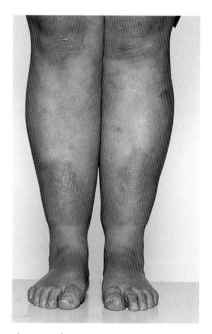

Figure 77b

Case 78

A 40-year-old gentleman presented as an emergency to the casualty department with increasing dyspnoea. On examination he was noted to have a right-sided neck mass.

A chest radiograph was performed (Figure 78a).

78.1 What is seen?

78.2 How else can this condition present?

A further radiological examination was then requested (Figure 78b).

78.3 What is this investigation and what does it show?

78.4 What is the natural history of this disease?

An operation was performed and the specimen is shown in Figure 78c.

78.5 What features are evident?

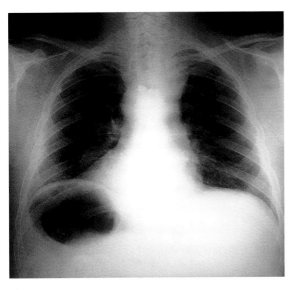

Figure 78a

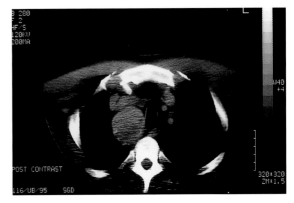

Figure 78b

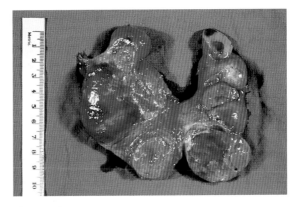

Figure 78c

Case 79

A 75-year-old lady presented with a short history of hoarseness and the development of a neck mass (Figure 79a).

79.1 What is evident on examination?

79.2 What are the common pathologies?

A second patient is shown undergoing a diagnostic procedure (Figures 79b and 79c).

79.3 What is being carried out and what is the diagnosis?

79.4 How are such lesions treated?

79.5 What is the prognosis of each?

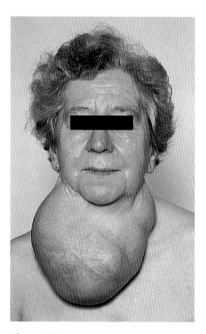

Figure 79a

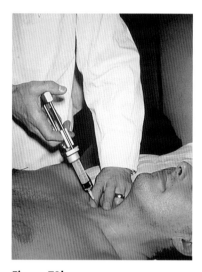

Figure 79b

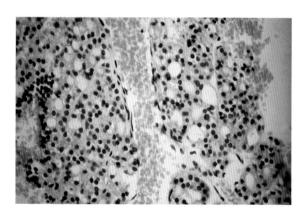

Figure 79c

Case 80

A 30-year-old gentleman underwent investigation following several admissions with renal colic. Biochemical
investigations revealed a calcium of 3.2 mmol/L and a
parathyroid hormone level of 450 pmol/L.

80.1 What is the diagnosis and what are the classical
presenting symptoms?

A radiological investigation was performed (Figure 80a).

80.2 What is seen?

80.3 What is the usual pathology?

80.4 What are the important complications of the
operation and what are the results of surgery?

A second patient underwent a repeat operation (Figure
80b).

80.5 What is seen in this operative photograph?

Case 81

A 30-year-old woman was admitted for investigation of
poorly controlled hypertension.

A 24 hour urine examination revealed a VMA of 15 mg,
metanephrines of 1.7 mg and a catecholamine level of
150 μg.

81.1 What is the diagnosis?

A radiological investigation was performed (Figure 81a).

81.2 What is the investigation and what is the diagnosis?

81.3 What are the principles of peri-operative management?

The specimen is shown in Figure 81b.

81.4 What features are evident?

81.5 What other causes of hypertension are amenable
to surgical treatment?

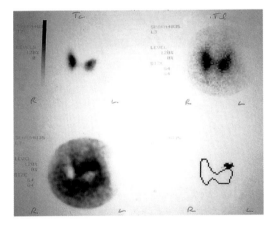

Figure 80a

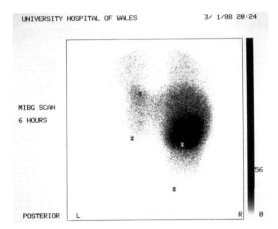

Figure 81a

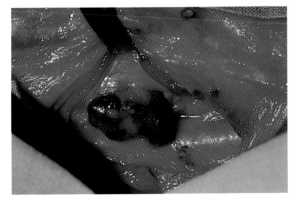

Figure 80b

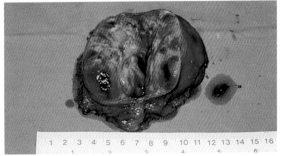

Figure 81b

Case 82

A 30-year-old gentleman was admitted for endocrine investigations (Figure 82a).

82.1 What features are evident on inspection of the abdomen?

82.2 What is the cause of this condition?

82.3 How may the diagnosis be confirmed?

A radiological investigation was performed (Figure 82b).

82.4 What does it show?

82.5 How should this condition be treated?

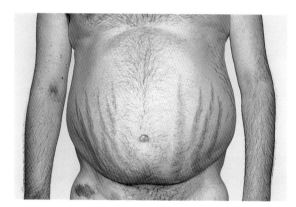

Figure 82a

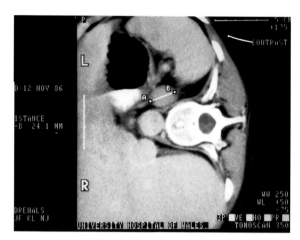

Figure 82b

Head and neck

Case 83

A 50-year-old gentleman presented to the outpatient clinic with a slow growing swelling over his left mandible (Figure 83a).

83.1 What is the differential and what is the likely diagnosis?

83.2 What common pathologies are encountered and what are their important features?

83.3 How may the diagnosis be confirmed?

83.4 How should such a lesion be treated and what are the important post-operative complications?

A 60-year-old woman presented with a similar lesion (Figure 83b).

83.5 What is seen and what is the probable diagnosis?

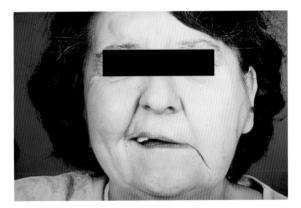

Figure 83b

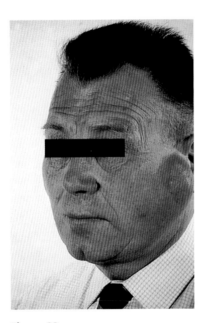

Figure 83a

Case 84

A 40-year-old gentleman presented with a painful swelling beneath his left mandible (Figure 84a).

84.1 What is the likely diagnosis and what is the differential?

A radiological investigation was performed (Figure 84b).

84.2 What is seen?

84.3 What is the demography of this condition?

84.4 How is this condition treated?

84.5 What structures are at risk during this operation?

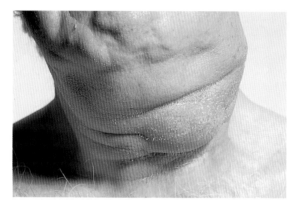

Figure 84a

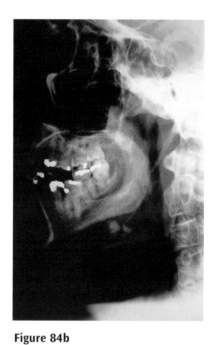

Figure 84b

Case 85

A 60-year-old gentleman presented with a large firm mass on the right side of his neck (Figure 85a).

85.1 What is the differential diagnosis?

On examination the mass was believed to be a group of enlarged lymph nodes.

85.2 What are the common causes of cervical lymphadenopathy?

85.3 What other investigations should be performed?

85.4 How should this patient be managed?

A woman from the Indian Subcontinent presented with a similar condition (Figure 85b).

85.5 What is the likely diagnosis?

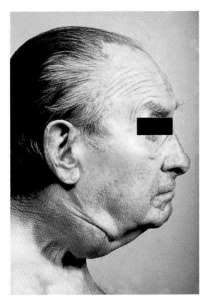

Figure 85a

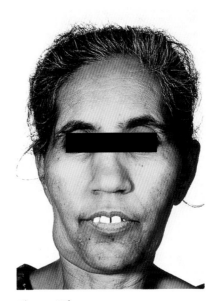

Figure 85b

Case 86

A 50-year-old gentleman presented with a midline neck swelling (Figures 86a and 86b).

86.1 What is the diagnosis?

86.2 What is the underlying defect?

86.3 What other conditions share the same aetiology?

86.4 What investigation must be performed prior to surgery?

86.5 How should the patient be managed?

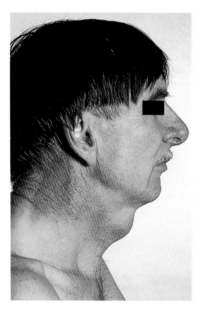

Figure 86a

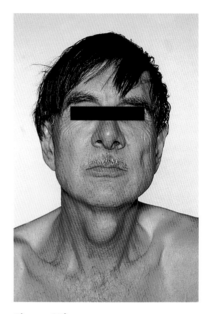

Figure 86b

Case 87

A 12-year-old girl presented with a soft swelling on the right side of her neck medial to sternocleidomastoid (Figure 87a).

87.1 What is the diagnosis?

87.2 What is the embryology of this condition?

87.3 What are the long-term sequelae if untreated?

87.4 What are the principles of operative treatment and what are the important complications?

A second patient attended the clinic with a small defect in the same anatomical region (Figure 87b).

87.5 What is the likely diagnosis?

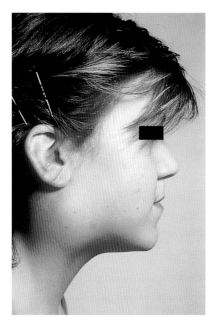

Figure 87a

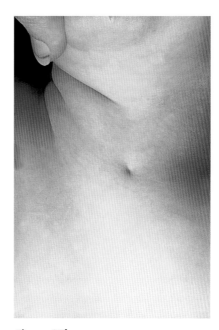

Figure 87b

Vascular

Case 88

The patient is an 80-year-old male smoker who on examination is found to have a pulsatile swelling in the abdomen.

88.1 What investigations are shown (Figures 88a–d) and what is seen in the per-operative picture in Figure 88e?

88.2 What are the risk factors for this condition?

88.3 What are the complications of this condition?

88.4 What factor is helpful in predicting the likelihood of the most common complication of this condition?

88.5 What are the morbidity and mortality of surgical treatment for this condition?

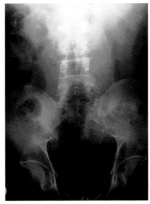

Figure 88a

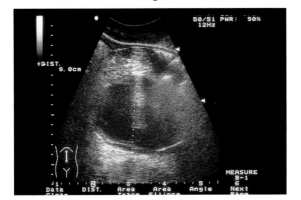

Figure 88b

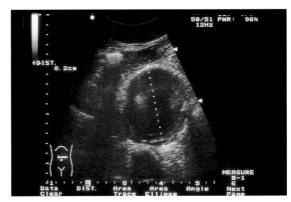

Figure 88c

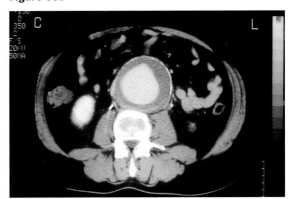

Figure 88d

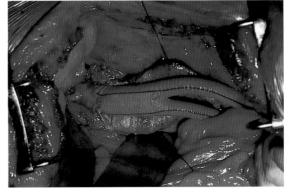

Figure 88e

Case 89

A 50-year-old female presents to the outpatient clinic with the problem indicated in Figures 89a and 89b.

89.1 What is the most likely diagnosis for the condition indicated in Figures 89a and 89b?

89.2 What are the other possible aetiologies of this condition?

89.3 What is the pathogenesis of this condition?

89.4 Figure 89c shows treatment of the condition indicated in Figures 89a and 89b. What is this treatment and how often should it be applied?

89.5 Figures 89d and 89e show another complication of this condition. What is the complication and what is its treatment?

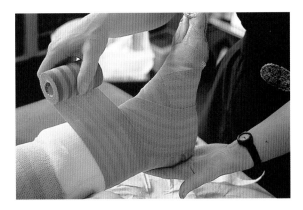

Figure 89c

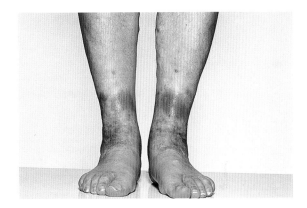

Figure 89d

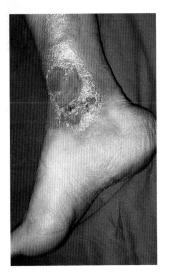

Figure 89a

Figure 89b

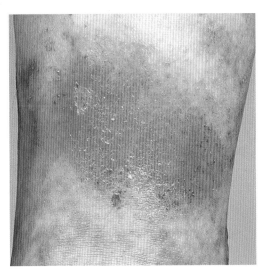

Figure 89e

Case 90

A 68-year-old male smoker has experienced transient dysphasia on several occasions. Treatment of the underlying problem was by an operation shown in Figures 90a and 90b.

90.1 What operation is being performed?

90.2 What are the indications for this operation? Justify your answer.

90.3 What investigations are undertaken pre-operatively?

90.4 What anatomical landmark is used as a reference when making the skin incision for this operation? What two operative details are sources of controversy?

90.5 What are the complications of this operation?

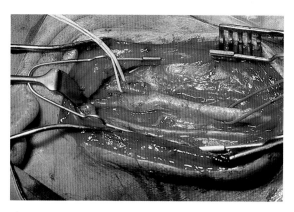

Figure 90a

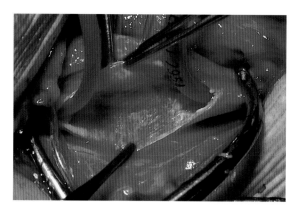

Figure 90b

Case 91

A patient who has been attending the rheumatology clinic for a number of years develops a new problem, indicated in Figures 91a and 91b. The two images were obtained at different times.

91.1 What is the diagnosis?

91.2 Give a description of the classical presentation of this disease?

91.3 Who is affected by this condition and what occupational factors may be implicated?

91.4 What systemic diseases may be seen in association?

91.5 What is the treatment of this condition?

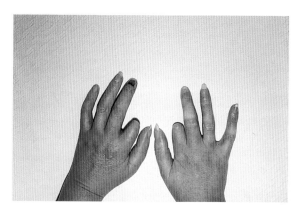

Figure 91a

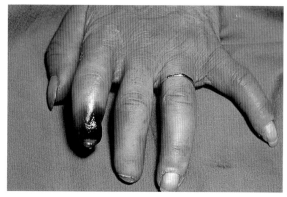

Figure 91b

Case 92

The young male indicated in Figures 92a and 92b has a commonly encountered surgical condition.

92.1 What is the diagnosis?

92.2 What particular fact should be elicited from the clinical history in a patient with this condition?

92.3 What are the indications for surgery?

92.4 Describe the surgical treatment of this condition.

92.5 What are the complications of surgical treatment of this condition?

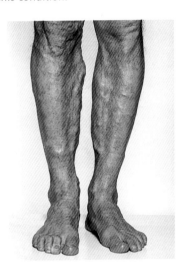

Figure 92a

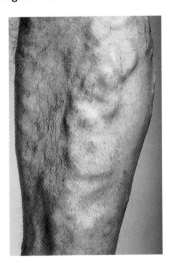

Figure 92b

Case 93

Figure 93 is a CT scan through the neck at the level of the carotid bifurcation.

93.1 What is the diagnosis?

93.2 What are the presenting features of this condition?

93.3 What is the differential diagnosis on clinical examination?

93.4 What are the epidemiology and aetiology of this condition?

93.5 What is the treatment of this condition?

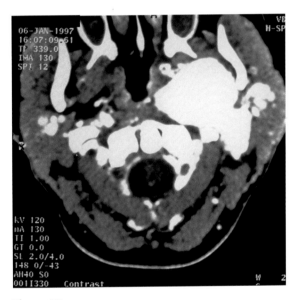

Figure 93

Case 94

Figures 94a–d are from four patients with the same underlying abnormality affecting two distinct anatomic sites.

94.1 What features are indicated in Figure 94a. What are the other causes of this?

94.2 What is shown in Figure 94b and what is its aetiology?

94.3 What condition is shown in Figures 94c and 94d, and what is its aetiology?

94.4 What may be associated with these abnormalities?

94.5 What are the main complications of these conditions?

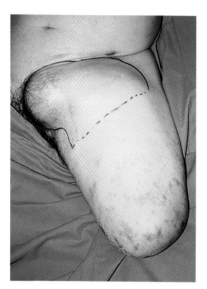

Figure 94a

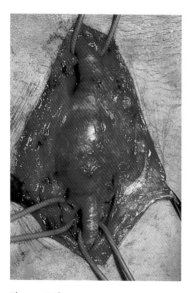

Figure 94b

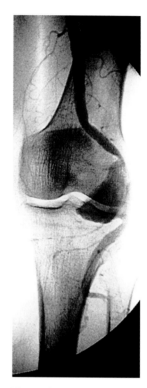

Figure 94c

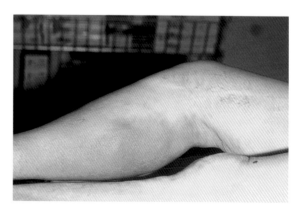

Figure 94d

Case 95

A 53-year-old female who has undergone right hemi-colectomy 2 weeks earlier develops acute onset pleuritic-type chest pain whilst convalescing from surgery at home.

95.1 What investigation is shown in Figure 95 and what is the abnormality?

95.2 What may be seen on chest radiography and electrocardiography?

95.3 What are the risk factors for the development of this condition?

95.4 What is the treatment of this condition?

95.5 Are there any preventative measures that can be taken in surgical patients?

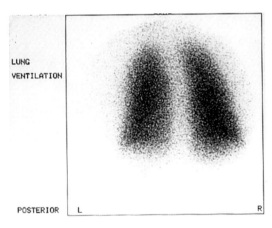

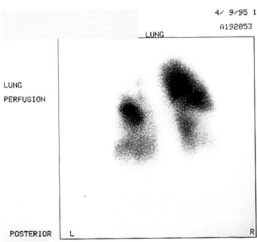

Figure 95

Case 96

A chronic medical condition underlies the problems seen in the patients shown in Figures 96a–c.

96.1 What is the medical problem?

96.2 What complication(s) of the medical problem cause these problems?

96.3 What are the principles of surgery for this condition?

96.4 How should patients with this medical problem undergoing surgery be managed?

96.5 What commonly prescribed medications may result in the development of this condition as a side-effect?

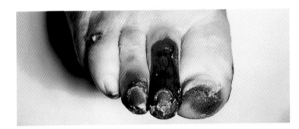

Figure 96a

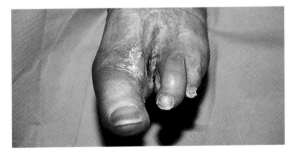

Figure 96b

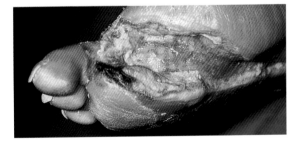

Figure 96c

Case 97

Figures 97a–c are taken from patients attending the vascular outpatient clinic with similar symptomatologies.

97.1 What investigations are shown (Figures 97a–c) and what are the abnormalities?

97.2 What is the typical presentation of patients with these radiographic appearances?

97.3 What is meant by Leriche's syndrome?

97.4 What is the treatment of the condition shown in Figures 97a and 97b?

97.5 What is the main cause of morbidity and mortality in this patient population? What other measures might be recommended?

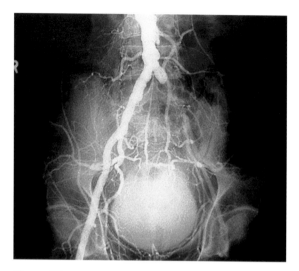

Figure 97a

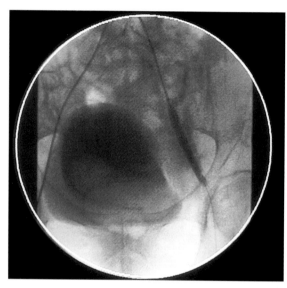

Figure 97c

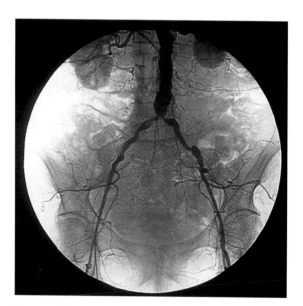

Figure 97b

Case 98

Figure 98a is from a patient with a condition being treated (in a different patient) in Figure 98b by use of a material indicated in Figure 98c.

98.1 What is indicated in Figures 98a–c?

98.2 What are the presenting features of this condition and what is meant by the term 'critical ischaemia'?

98.3 Explain what is meant by an ankle-brachial index, stating what the normal value is and how it is altered in disease states.

98.4 For the operation indicated in Figure 98b, use of what conduit results in the best long-term patency rate? If this preferred conduit is used, the operation may be performed in one of two ways. Describe them and comment on their relative merits.

98.5 What other conduits may be used?

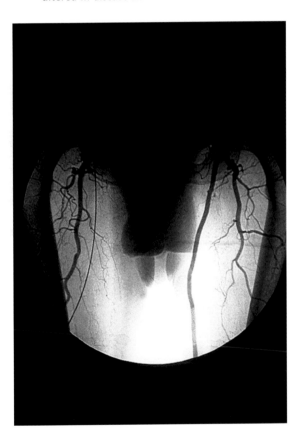

Figure 98a

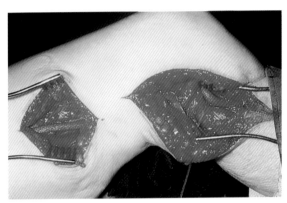

Figure 98b

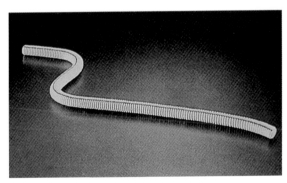

Figure 98c

Case 99

Figures 99a–e indicate the same condition in the upper (Figures 99a–c) and lower (Figures 99d and 99e) limbs.

99.1 What is the diagnosis? What do you think is the likely aetiology of the appearance seen in Figure 99a?

99.2 What are the presenting features of this condition?

99.3 What is the origin of this condition?

99.4 What is the main differential diagnosis?

99.5 What is the treatment of this condition?

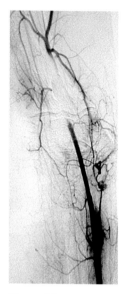

Figure 99c

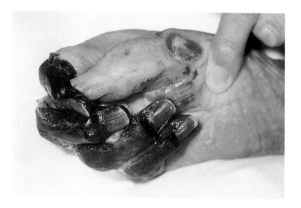

Figure 99a

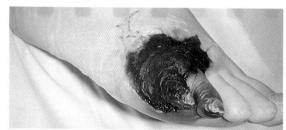

Figure 99d

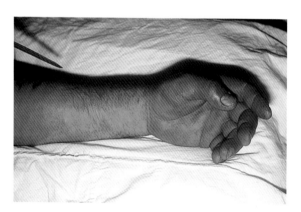

Figure 99b

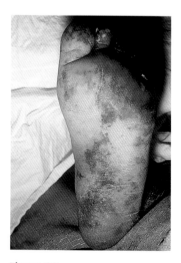

Figure 99e

Case 100

A 60-year-old gentleman with end-stage renal disease was admitted for a routine operation (Figure 100a).

100.1 What procedure is being performed in Figure 100a?

100.2 What are the early complications of this operation?

100.3 What other therapeutic options are available?

100.4 The patient later returned with a complication of surgery (Figure 100b). What is seen and what is the pathogenesis?

100.5 What is demonstrated in Figure 100c and how is this complication managed?

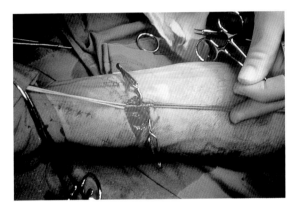

Figure 100a

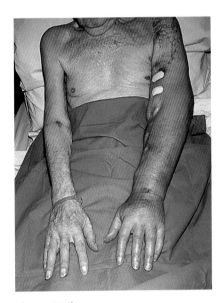

Figure 100b

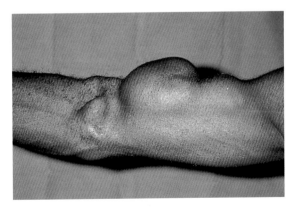

Figure 100c

Paediatric

Case 101

A baby boy presented with a large soft mass on the right side of his neck (Figure 101).

101.1 What is the diagnosis?

101.2 What clinical test is diagnostic of the condition?

101.3 What is the underlying cause?

101.4 How is this condition managed?

101.5 Are there any long-term sequelae if left untreated?

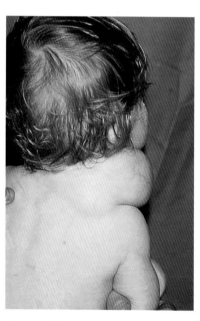

Figure 101

Case 102

A male infant was referred with a prominent peri-umbilical swelling (Figure 102a).

102.1 What is the likely diagnosis?

102.2 How common is this condition?

102.3 What defect is responsible for this condition?

102.4 Is an operation required?

A second patient with a small erythematous swelling also attended the clinic (Figure 102b).

102.5 What is the diagnosis?

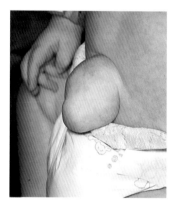

Figure 102a

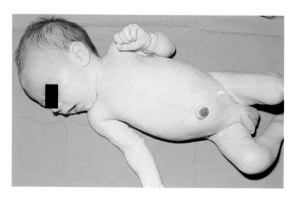

Figure 102b

Case 103

Two newborn infants were referred with different abdominal wall defects (Figures 103a and 103b).

103.1 What are the diagnoses?

103.2 What is the pathogenesis of these two conditions?

103.3 How may the two conditions be distinguished clinically?

103.4 What are the principles of management?

103.5 What is the prognosis of the two conditions?

Case 104

A newborn boy was rushed from the delivery suite to the special care baby unit and a surgical opinion requested.

A radiograph was requested (Figure 104).

104.1 What diagnostic feature is evident?

104.2 What would be found on examination?

104.3 What is the underlying defect?

104.4 How is the condition treated?

104.5 What factors determine the prognosis?

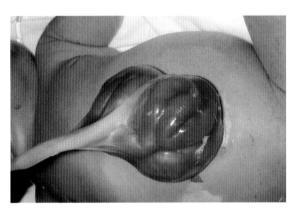

Figure 103a

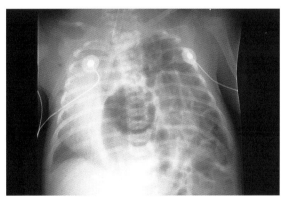

Figure 104

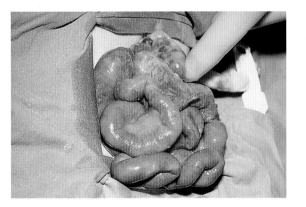

Figure 103b

Case 105

A 6-week-old baby presented as an emergency with projectile vomiting.

105.1 What is the likely diagnosis?

105.2 What are the characteristic demographics?

A radiological contrast study was performed (Figure 105a).

105.3 What features are evident?

105.4 What are the characteristic biochemical abnormalities associated with this condition?

An operation was performed (Figure 105b).

105.5 What is seen?

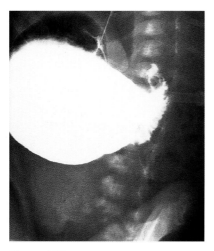

Figure 105a

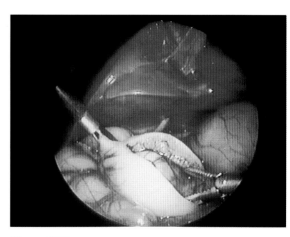

Figure 105b

Case 106

A 5-year-old boy was admitted as an emergency with colicky abdominal pain, vomiting and the passage of redcurrant jelly stools.

106.1 What is the probable diagnosis and what are the common aetiological factors?

A radiologic investigation was performed (Figure 106a).

106.2 What is seen?

A contrast study was then performed (Figure 106b).

106.3 What is seen and why is this investigation chosen?

He underwent a laparotomy and the findings are shown (Figure 106c).

106.4 What is seen?

This patient had characteristic facies of a less common cause of this condition (Figure 106d).

106.5 What is the diagnosis?

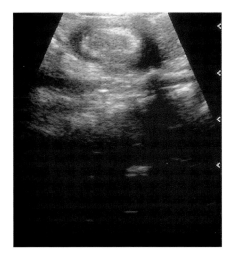

Figure 106a

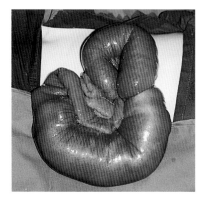

Figure 106c

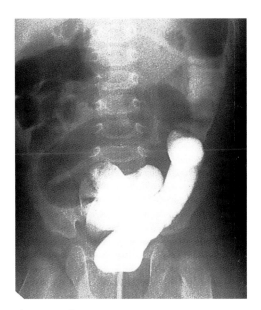

Figure 106b

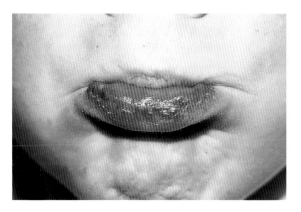

Figure 106d

Case 107

A male neonate presented with an inability to swallow his feeds.

A plain chest radiograph was performed (Figure 107a).

107.1 What is the diagnostic feature?

A second patient presented with a similar condition and a contrast study was performed (Figure 107b).

107.2 What is seen and how is this condition classified?

107.3 What treatment options are available?

Examination of the perineum revealed a second anomaly (Figure 107c).

107.4 What is seen and what other features may be present as part of a syndrome?

107.5 How is this anomaly managed?

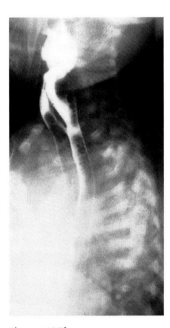

Figure 107b

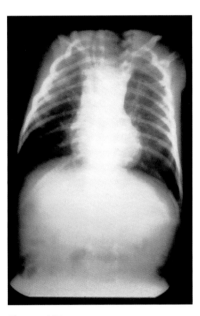

Figure 107a

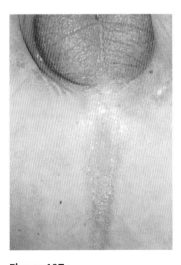

Figure 107c

Case 108

A female neonate with abdominal distension and bilious vomiting was referred for a surgical opinion.

108.1   What diagnostic feature is evident?

An abdominal radiograph was performed (Figure 108a).

108.2   What is the aetiology of this condition?

108.3   How is this condition classified?

108.4   Are there any important associations?

The child underwent a laparotomy (Figure 108b).

108.5   What is seen?

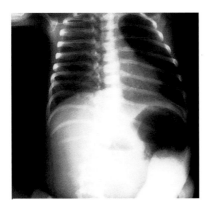

Figure 108a

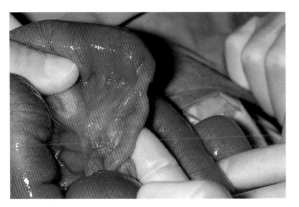

Figure 108b

Case 109

A premature infant was referred with abdominal distension (Figure 109a).

109.1   What feature is evident on clinical examination?

109.2   What are the important differential diagnoses?

A plain abdominal radiograph was performed.

109.3   What sign is evident and what is the diagnosis?

109.4   What are the important aetiological factors?

109.5   How is the condition treated and what is the outcome?

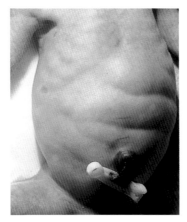

Figure 109a

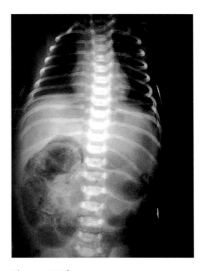

Figure 109b

Case 110

A 12-year-old boy presented to the outpatient department with a large left-sided abdominal mass.

110.1 What are the important differential diagnoses?

An intravenous urogram was performed (Figure 110a)

110.2 What does it show?

A second patient presented with a similar condition and a CT of the abdomen was performed (Figure 110b).

110.3 What is seen?

110.4 What other investigations are required pre-operatively?

110.5 How should this condition be managed?

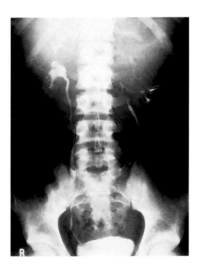

Figure 110a

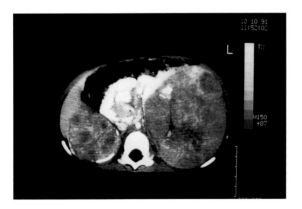

Figure 110b

Case 111

A 2-year-old boy attended the outpatient clinic following an observation made on his genitalia (Figure 111).

111.1 What is the most likely diagnosis?

111.2 Can these conditions be distinguished clinically?

111.3 What radiological investigations may be of use?

111.4 How is this condition treated?

111.5 What are the important long-term sequelae if the condition is not treated?

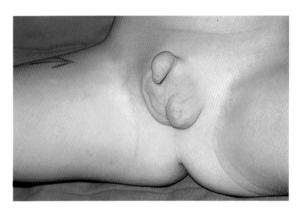

Figure 111

Case 112

An infant presented to the paediatric outpatients with a lump in his perineum (Figure 112).

112.1 What is the diagnosis?

112.2 What is the pathogenesis?

112.3 Where else may these 'lumps' occur?

112.4 Is testicular development normal in this condition?

112.5 How should this case be treated?

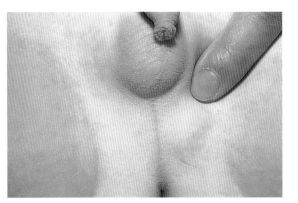

Figure 112

Case 113

A 6-year-old boy presented with a painful non-retractile foreskin (Figure 113a).

113.1 What is seen and what is the diagnosis?

113.2 What is the underlying defect?

113.3 How is this condition treated?

113.4 What are the other indications for this operation?

A second patient had a less severe form of the condition.

113.5 What procedure is being performed in Figure 113b?

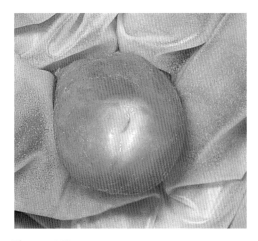

Figure 113a

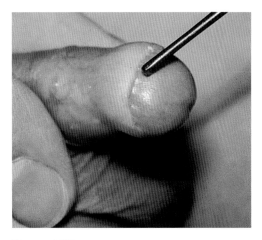

Figure 113b

Case 114

A young boy was admitted as an emergency with a discoloured left hemiscrotum (Figure 114a).

114.1 What is the differential diagnosis?

An emergency operation was performed (Figure 114b).

114.2 What is seen?

114.3 What are the recognised aetiological factors?

114.4 What are the principles of this operation?

A second patient was admitted with similar symptomatology but a different underlying disease (Figure 114c).

114.5 What is the diagnosis?

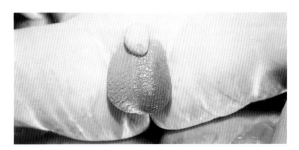

Figure 114a

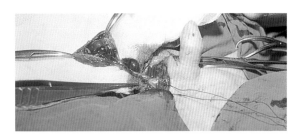

Figure 114b

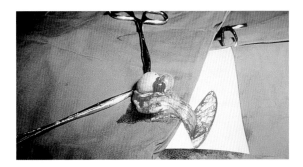

Figure 114c

Case 115

A 4-year-old boy presented with a painless lump in his right groin which increased in size on crying (Figure 115a).

115.1 What is the diagnosis?

115.2 How common is this condition?

115.3 What is the underlying defect?

115.4 Do all children with this condition require surgery?

115.5 What operation is being performed in Figure 115b?

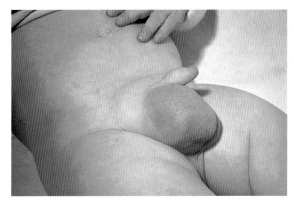

Figure 115a

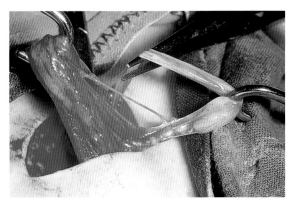

Figure 115b

Urology

Case 116

Figures 116a and 116b are from two different patients with the same underlying condition.

116.1 What is shown in Figures 116a and 116b, and what is the diagnosis?

116.2 What are the presenting features of this disease?

116.3 What are the investigations of choice for the symptom that this condition most commonly causes?

116.4 What is the aetiology of this condition?

116.5 What is the treatment of this condition?

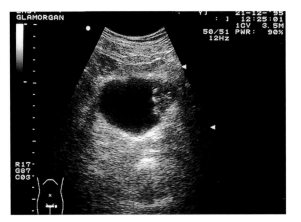

Figure 116a

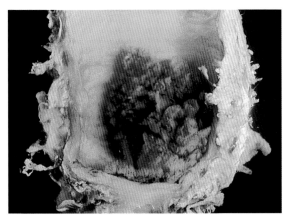

Figure 116b

Case 117

A 75-year-old male presents with a 3 month history of haematuria and loin pain.

117.1 What investigation is shown in Figure 117a and what is the diagnosis confirmed by the specimen indicated in Figure 117b?

117.2 Describe the presenting features of this condition.

117.3 Outline the surgical treatment of this condition.

117.4 What is shown in Figure 117c? Neoplasia of which other organ results in a similar phenomenon?

117.5 What neoplasm affecting the organ seen in Figure 117b occurs in patients with tuberous sclerosis?

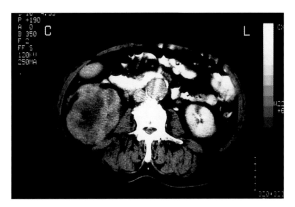

Figure 117a

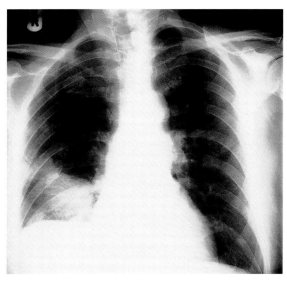

Figure 117c

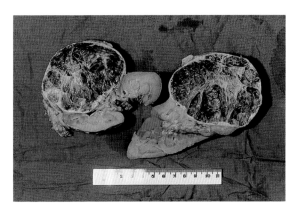

Figure 117b

Case 118

A 36-year-old male has noticed that his left testis has increased in size? Figure 118 shows the macroscopic appearance of the testis following surgery.

118.1 What is the most likely diagnosis?

118.2 How does this condition usually present?

118.3 Are biochemical markers useful in monitoring this patient? Justify your answer.

118.4 What are the principles of surgical treatment?

118.5 If the patient was a male over the age of 60 years, what would the most likely diagnosis be?

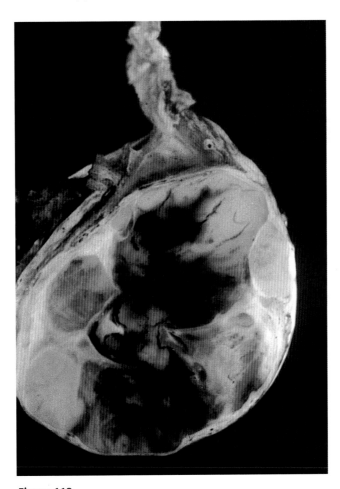

Figure 118

Case 119

A 73-year-old male attends the outpatient clinic with an 18 month history of increasing difficulty passing urine. Biochemical investigations reveal a prostate-specific antigen level of 4 ng/mL.

119.1 What is shown in Figure 119a? What may be performed at the time of the procedure?

119.2 What investigations would you request on this patient? What would you consider as indications for surgery?

119.3 What is shown in Figures 119b and 119c?

119.4 What are the complications of this operation?

119.5 If this gentleman had been catheterised for the 2 months pre-operatively, what complication would he be more at risk of and how could it be prevented?

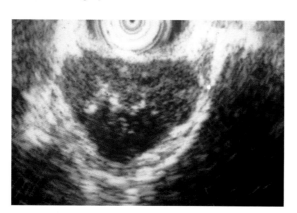

Figure 119a

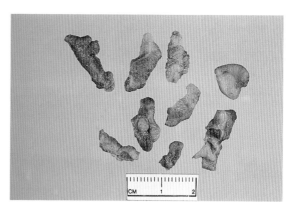

Figure 119c

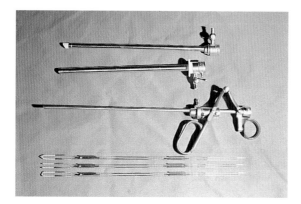

Figure 119b

Case 120

The patient is a 68-year-old male who has developed urinary frequency, hesitancy, nocturia and a poor urinary flow over the last 3 months. His prostate-specific antigen is 151 ng/mL.

120.1 What is the most likely diagnosis?

120.2 What investigations are shown (Figures 120a–d) and what is demonstrated?

120.3 Is this gentleman amenable to curative surgery? Should he have an operation? If yes, what?

120.4 What is the treatment of this condition, for this gentleman and in general?

120.5 What is the epidemiology of this condition?

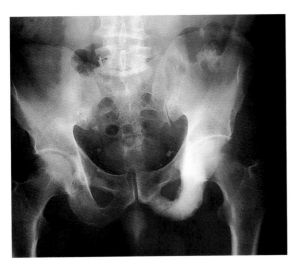

Figure 120a

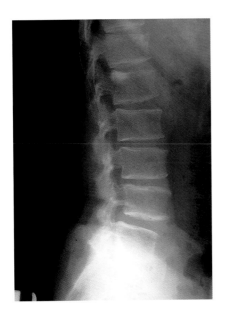

Figure 120b

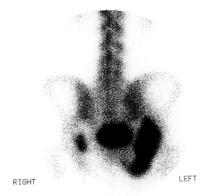

Figure 120c

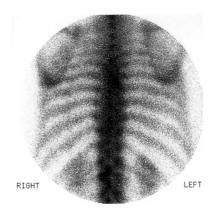

Figure 120d

Case 121

A middle-aged male attends an outpatient clinic with a scrotal swelling indicated in Figures 121a and 121b.

121.1 Is this lump likely to be painful?

121.2 How does one determine the nature of a scrotal swelling?

121.3 What is the likely diagnosis?

121.4 What is the treatment?

121.5 What is the main complication of surgical treatment for this condition?

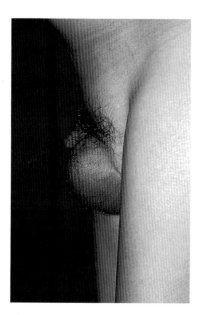

Figure 121a

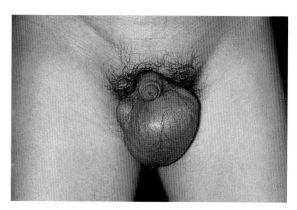

Figure 121b

Case 122

The patient, a male aged 46 years, has experienced recurrent episodes of loin pain for the last 12 months.

122.1 What investigation is shown (Figures 122a–c) and what is indicated?

122.2 How should this condition be managed?

122.3 What is the likely chemical composition of the underlying cause?

122.4 What is the epidemiology of this condition?

122.5 What medical conditions predispose to the development of this condition?

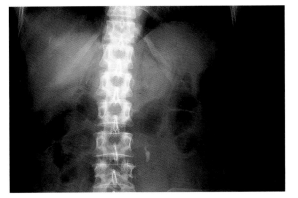

Figure 122a

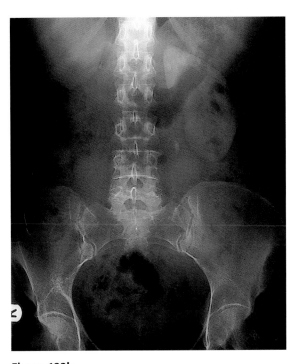

Figure 122b

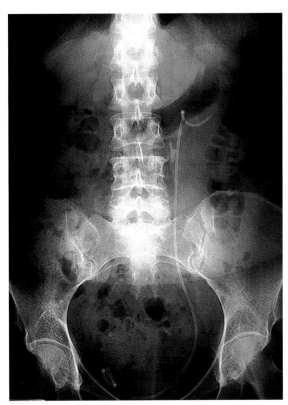

Figure 122c

Case 123

A 20-year-old male attends the outpatient clinic with the scrotal lump seen in Figure 123.

123.1 What is the diagnosis?

123.2 Which side is more commonly affected?

123.3 Who develops this condition?

123.4 What symptoms may result from this problem?

123.5 What is the treatment of this condition?

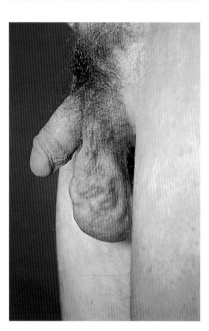

Figure 123

Case 124

A 64-year-old male with a 3 month history of haematuria has undergone an investigation (Figure 124).

124.1 What is the investigation and how is it performed? What other investigation will image the same region?

124.2 What is the abnormality and most likely diagnosis?

124.3 What is the epidemiology of this condition?

124.4 What is the treatment of this condition?

124.5 Following successful treatment what is this patient at risk of subsequently? Expand on your answer.

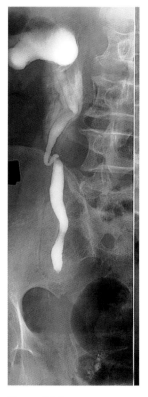

Figure 124

Case 125

Figure 125 shows the post-mortem appearances of an organ affected by an inherited condition.

125.1 What is the diagnosis?

125.2 What are the genetics of this condition?

125.3 What are the systemic features of this condition?

125.4 How does this condition usually present? At what age?

125.5 How common is this condition amongst patients receiving treatment for end-stage disease of this organ? What is the surgical relevance of this condition?

Case 126

A 50-year-old male has developed the condition seen in Figure 126a following an operation.

126.1 What is the diagnosis?

126.2 What is the cause of this condition?

126.3 What is the treatment?

126.4 When the condition was first described, which patient group was affected and how does that differ from the pattern seen nowadays?

126.5 Figure 126b shows a similar process affecting a different region of the body. By what name is this condition known and what name is given to a similar condition affecting the abdominal wall?

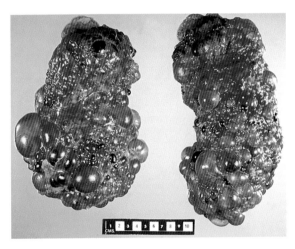

Figure 125

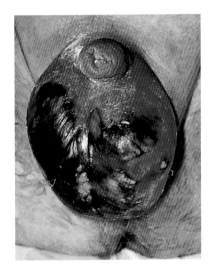

Figure 126a

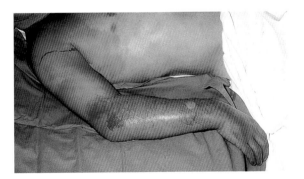

Figure 126b

Case 127

A 34-year-old gentleman with chronic renal failure underwent a cadaveric renal transplant.

127.1 What are the important early post-operative complications?

127.2 What complications are shown in Figures 127a and 127b and what is their common aetiology?

A patient who had undergone a successful operation 6 months previously underwent investigation for poorly controlled hypertension (Figures 127c and 127d).

127.3 What is seen in Figure 127c and what has been carried out in Figure 127d?

This patient later presented with abdominal pain and a CT scan (Figure 127e) was performed.

127.4 What is seen?

127.5 What are the results of renal transplantation?

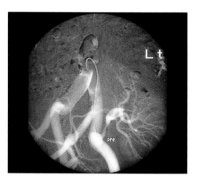

Figure 127c

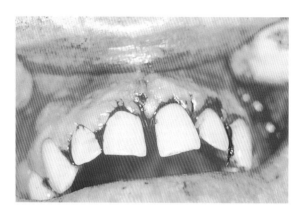

Figure 127a

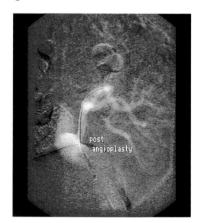

Figure 127d

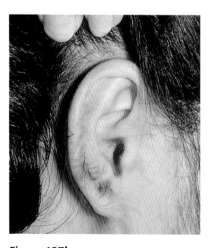

Figure 127b

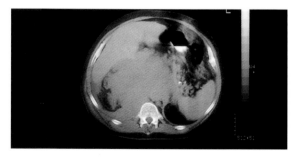

Figure 127e

Orthopaedics and trauma

Case 128

The clinical (Figure 128a) and radiographic (Figure 128b) appearances of a common upper limb injury are shown. Figure 128c shows the radiographic appearance of a similar type of injury to a different part of the upper limb.

128.1 What injuries are shown in Figures 128a–c?

128.2 How are they treated?

128.3 What are the early complications?

128.4 What are the late complications?

128.5 What are the other forms of this type of injury to the joint affected in Figures 128a and 128b?

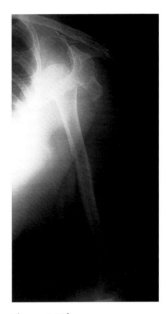

Figure 128b

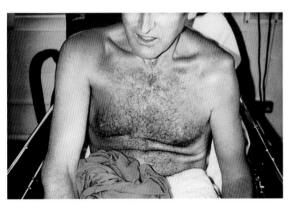

Figure 128a

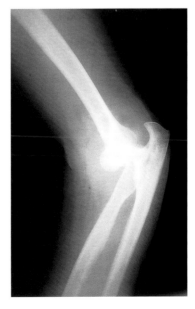

Figure 128c

Case 129

Figures 129a and 129b show a similar injury in a child (Figure 129a) and an adult (Figure 129b). Figure 129c shows a different injury in an elderly female patient.

129.1 What injuries are shown in Figures 129a–c?

129.2 What are the complications of the injury shown in Figures 129a and 129b?

129.3 How should the injury be treated?

129.4 Whose classification is commonly used to describe the injury shown in Figure 129c?

129.5 What is the treatment of this injury?

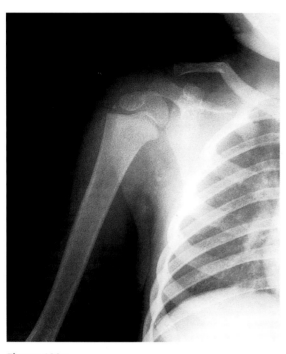

Figure 129a

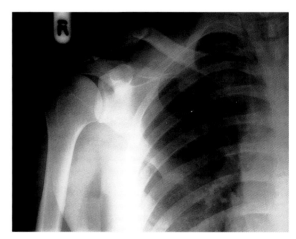

Figure 129b

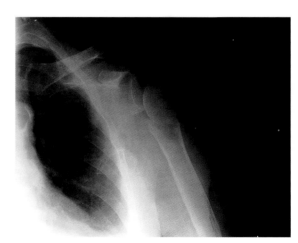

Figure 129c

Case 130

Figure 130a is a radiograph of a 25-year-old footballer following an ankle injury. Figures 130b and 130c are clinical (130b) and radiographic (130c) images of an ankle injury in a 68-year-old female.

130.1 What is indicated in Figures 130a–c?

130.2 Is the injury shown in Figure 130a the most usual ankle injury? How are ankle ligament injuries treated?

130.3 Give the commonly used classification of ankle fractures. How is it helpful?

130.4 What are the complications of ankle fractures?

130.5 What is of particular consideration in the patient indicated by Figures 130b and 130c?

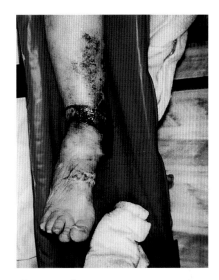

Figure 130b

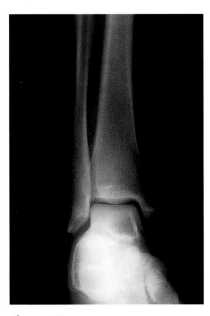

Figure 130a

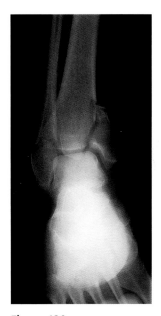

Figure 130c

Case 131

Figures 131a–c are illustrative examples of the methods of managing three different long bone fractures.

131.1 For each patient state which long bone(s) have been injured and how the fractures have been managed.

131.2 What are the local and systemic complications of long bone fractures? Divide your answer into early and late.

131.3 What treatment method, not shown, may be used to treat open fractures?

131.4 What classification of open fractures is commonly used? Give the classification. What is its usefulness?

131.5 What is meant by a stress fracture?

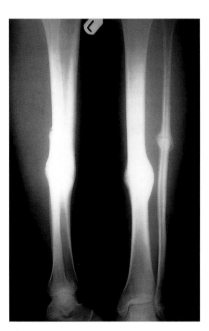

Figure 131a

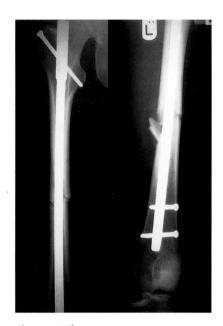

Figure 131b

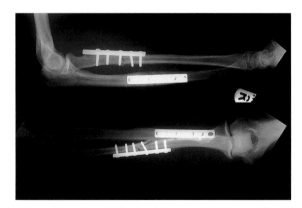

Figure 131c

Case 132

The patient is a 78-year-old patient from a nursing home attending the Accident and Emergency Department following a trivial fall (Figures 132a and 132b).

132.1   What is the diagnosis?

132.2   Who is affected by this condition?

132.3   How is the injury classified? Give the classification.

132.4   What are the complications specific to this injury?

132.5   What is the management of this injury?

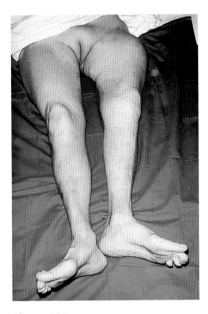

Figure 132a

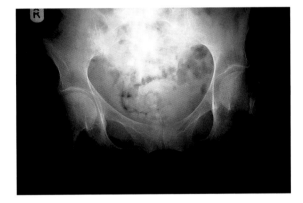

Figure 132b

Case 133

Figures 133a–d show different methods of treatment for fractures of the proximal femur.

133.1 What fixation devices have been used in Figures 133a–d?

133.2 What injuries are the devices in Figures 133c and 133d used to treat?

133.3 What other means of fracture fixation may be appropriate for the injury in Figure 133d? What is often associated with these fractures?

133.4 Aside from fractures of the proximal femur what fractures are a common cause of non-weight-bearing in the elderly, and how are they managed?

133.5 What is the management of a patient with hip pain but normal plain radiography?

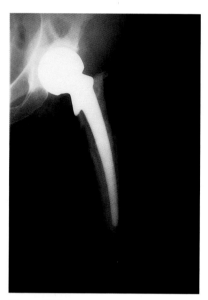

Figure 133a

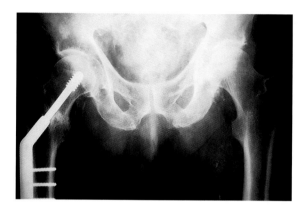

Figure 133c

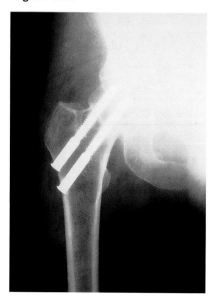

Figure 133b

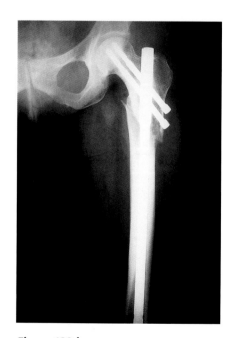

Figure 133d

Case 134

Figures 134a and 134b relate to a common injury seen in childhood. Figures 134c and 134d relate to an injury sustained by a female aged 45.

134.1 What injuries are shown in Figures 134a and 134c?

134.2 How have they been treated?

134.3 What are the complications of the injury shown in Figures 134a and 134b?

134.4 What are the complications of the injury shown in Figures 134c and 134d?

134.5 What are the clinical features and management of the most feared complication of the injury shown in Figures 134a and 134b?

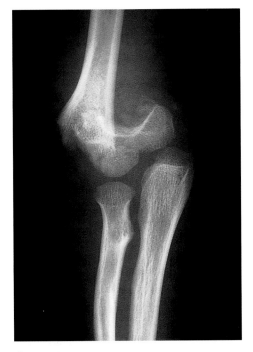

Figure 134a

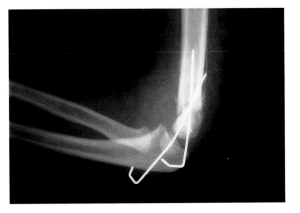

Figure 134b

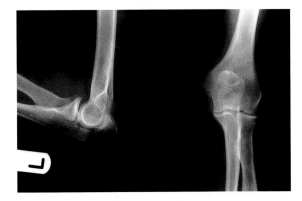

Figure 134c

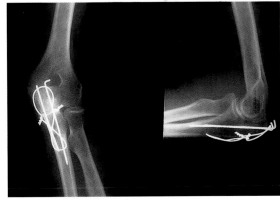

Figure 134d

Case 135

Figures 135a–c relate to injuries around the wrist joint. Figure 135a shows a very common injury in elderly female patients. Figure 135b shows an uncommon injury at this site and Figure 135c relates to a common injury seen in childhood.

135.1 What injuries are shown in Figures 135a–c?

135.2 What is the management of the injury shown in Figure 135a?

135.3 What injury might be confused with the injury shown in Figure 135b? What is the management of the injury shown in Figure 135b?

135.4 What are the complications of the injury shown in Figure 135a?

135.5 What is the treatment of the injury shown in Figure 135c?

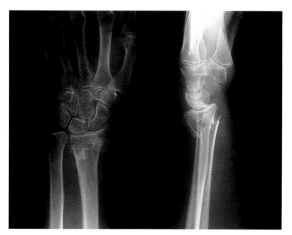

Figure 135a

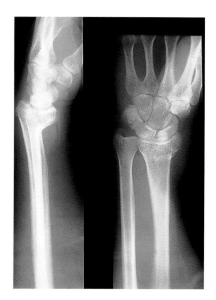

Figure 135b

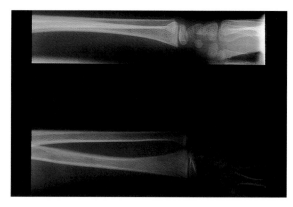

Figure 135c

Case 136

Figure 136 is a radiograph of a common carpal injury.

136.1 What is the injury? Imaging of the wrist in what position may highlight this injury?

136.2 Who is affected by this injury?

136.3 What is considered the diagnostic sign for this injury? What is the management of patients with this diagnostic sign but a normal radiograph?

136.4 What are the complications of this injury? What is the anatomical basis for them?

136.5 What is the management of this injury?

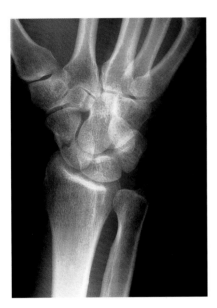

Figure 136

Case 137

Figures 137a and 137b are from two different patients in their early twenties with injuries affecting different regions of the same structure.

137.1 What abnormalities are shown?

137.2 What is the main complication of injuries such as this? What accident mechanisms result in these patterns of injury?

137.3 Is this radiograph (Figure 137a) satisfactory? Justify your answer.

137.4 How many people are required to log-roll a patient with these injuries?

137.5 Whose classification is useful in assessing the relative stability of these injuries? Give the classification?

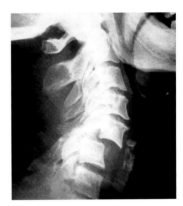

Figure 137a

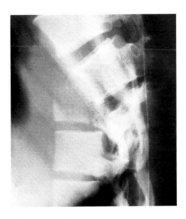

Figure 137b

Case 138

Figures 138a and 138b relate to injuries sustained by two young adults following their assault outside a nightclub. Figure 138c shows a complication of the injury sustained in Figure 138b.

138.1 What injuries are shown in Figures 138a–c and what imaging technique has been used in Figure 138c?

138.2 What method of assessing level of consciousness is commonly used? Give the classification? How is a severe head injury defined?

138.3 What are the indications for hospitalisation following a head injury?

138.4 What is meant by the term secondary brain injury?

138.5 What is an additional complication with base of skull fractures?

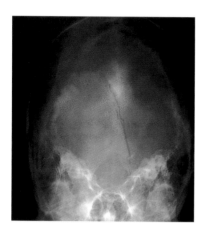

Figure 138a

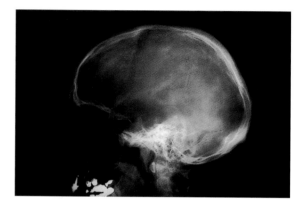

Figure 138b

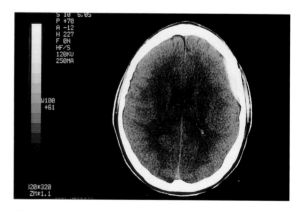

Figure 138c

Case 139

These two young adults sustained the injuries seen in Figures 139a and 139b whilst sleeping.

139.1 What is the likely cause of these injuries? How should these patients be managed?

139.2 What radiographs should be obtained initially on multiply injured patients?

139.3 What is meant by the term secondary survey?

139.4 Do these patients have a potential airway problem? Justify your answer indicating what features make this likely or unlikely.

139.5 What simple method is commonly used to assess the extent of injuries such as these? Can it be used for all patients? If not, who?

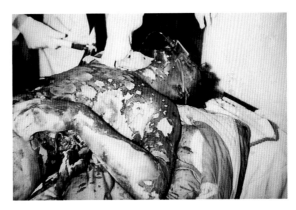

Figure 139b

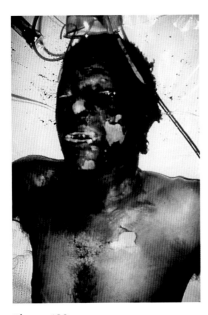

Figure 139a

Case 140

Figures 140a–c were obtained from three different patients sustaining injuries to the same area.

140.1 What is shown in Figures 140a–c? What is the likely injury mechanism of the patient shown in Figure 140a?

140.2 What is the abnormality shown in Figure 140b? Is this commonly seen on chest radiographs?

140.3 What are the clinical features of the condition shown in Figure 140b?

140.4 What are the indications for chest drain insertion in a trauma patient?

140.5 What cardiac problem may be seen following blunt or penetrating trauma to the thorax? How is it treated?

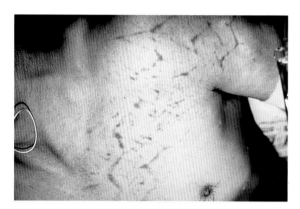

Figure 140a

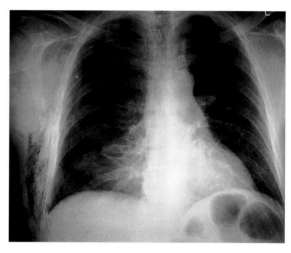

Figure 140c

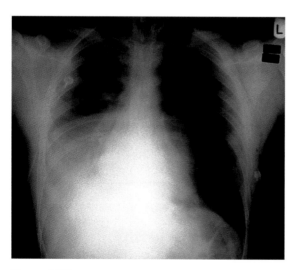

Figure 140b

Case 141

Following an injury sustained in a road traffic accident the patient has undergone laparotomy and an abdominal organ removed (Figure 141a).

141.1 What organ has been removed? What is shown in Figure 141b obtained from another patient with a similar problem? What injuries are commonly seen in association with this injury?

141.2 Describe the performance of peritoneal lavage? What indicates a positive result?

141.3 What are the indications for peritoneal lavage in a trauma patient?

141.4 The organ shown in Figure 141a is on occasions removed for other reasons. What are the other indications for removal of this organ?

141.5 What are the complications of removal of this organ?

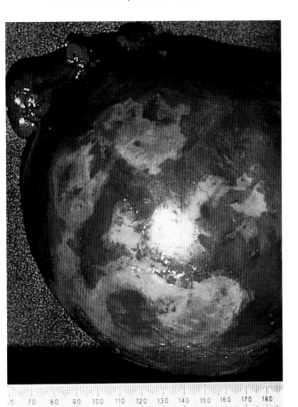

Figure 141b

Figure 141a

Case 142

The radiograph of a 71-year-old female with left hip pain is shown (Figure 142a). She subsequently underwent an operation. Figure 142b shows the radiographic appearance following surgery.

142.1 What do Figures 142a and 142b show? What medical condition underlies the observations?

142.2 What are the radiographic features of this condition?

142.3 What is the treatment of this condition (at this site)?

142.4 What are the complications of surgical treatment?

142.5 What are the predisposing factors for the development of this condition?

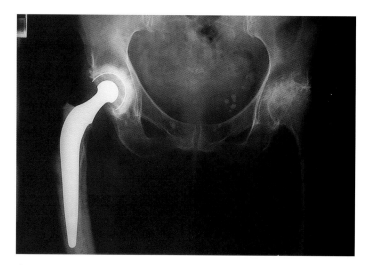

Figure 142a

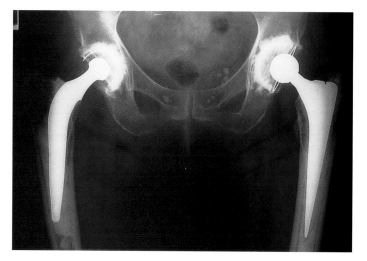

Figure 142b

Part II

Answers

General

Case 1 – Indirect inguinal hernia

1.1 Indirect inguinal hernia.

1.2 Inguinal hernias are common with 3% of the UK population undergoing herniorrhaphy, of whom 65% have indirect hernias. The peak age is 60 years and the ratio of males to females is 12:1.

1.3 The patient should undergo surgical repair. The current favoured procedures are:

  1 Shouldice repair in which the transversalis fascia is divided and double-breasted. Then the conjoined tendon is sutured to the iliopubic tract using non-absorbable sutures;

  2 Lichtenstein repair, in which a tension-free repair is performed by suturing a polypropylene mesh over the defect.

1.4 Complications include haematoma formation, seroma formation, infection, inadvertent damage to the ductus deferens, ischaemic orchitis, hydrocoele, urinary retention and recurrence. The mortality for elective repair is about 0.3% increasing to 6% for strangulated hernias.

1.5 This is a herniogram performed by injecting a small quantity of water-soluble contrast into the peritoneal cavity. The contrast demonstrates a large left-sided indirect hernia as seen clinically and also a small right indirect inguinal hernia.

Case 2 – Direct inguinal hernia

2.1 The differential diagnosis includes: inguinal hernia (direct and indirect), femoral hernia, saphena varix, lymph node, lipoma of cord, femoral aneurysm, psoas abscess, ectopic testis, hydrocoele of cord (canal of Nuck in women). In this case the likely diagnosis is a direct inguinal hernia.

2.2 Predisposing factors include cigarette smoking, chronic obstructive airways disease, heavy manual work and previous appendicectomy in which the ilio-inguinal nerve may have been damaged (right-sided hernias).

2.3 A weakening of the transversalis fascia in the posterior wall of the inguinal canal through a region known as Hesselbach's triangle. The medial boundary of this triangle is the rectus sheath, laterally are the inferior epigastric vessels and inferiorly is the inguinal ligament.

2.4 Inguinal hernias are said to arise above and medial to the pubic tubercle (femoral – below and lateral). Direct hernias are often difficult to distinguish pre-operatively from small indirect hernias, the distinction being often only possible at the time of repair.

2.5 The patient should undergo herniorrhaphy by either Shouldice or Lichtenstein methods.

Case 3 – Femoral hernia

3.1 The likely diagnosis is a femoral hernia. After inguinal hernia, this is the second most common type of hernia with a female predominance of 4:1.

3.2 The underlying cause is a weakness of the femoral ring secondary to atrophy or dilatation. With time the fascia transversalis is forced into the canal and may be followed by peritoneum and extraperitoneal fat giving the characteristic thick-walled feel of the hernia.

3.3 Several approaches are possible including crural (low), inguinal (high) and extraperitoneal. The extraperitoneal approach gives the most effective exposure and is recommended for strangulated hernias as it allows for reduction of the hernia, inspection of the bowel for signs of ischaemic damage (with access for bowel resection if required), and closure of the neck of the sac.

3.4 Important procedure-specific side-effects include: damage to an accessory obturator artery if present, bladder perforation and femoral vein stenosis.

3.5 The radiograph shows features of small bowel obstruction with dilated small bowel loops. Femoral hernias (together with adhesions and tumours) are one of the most common causes of small bowel obstruction in the Western world.

Case 4 – Paraumbilical hernia

4.1 Paraumbilical hernia.

4.2 The classic patient is an obese, multiparous middle-aged woman.

4.3 The hernia usually consists of omentum but may also contain either small or large bowel.

4.4 The hernia occurs due to a weakness in the linea alba either above or below the umbilicus. Large hernias containing bowel may cause gastrointestinal symptoms through traction on viscera.

4.5 Yes. Paraumbilical hernias have narrow necks and are prone to irreducibility, obstruction and strangulation.

Case 5 – Incisional hernia

5.1 Incisional hernia.

5.2 Factors predisposing to incisional hernias include: preoperative malnutrition (protein, vitamin C or zinc deficiency); jaundice; uraemia; respiratory disease (chronic obstructive airways disease, smoking); obesity; steroids; midline incisions; poor operative technique (excessive suture tension, incorrect suture material); post-operative distension; wound infection; haematoma.

5.3 Measures to reduce the incidence of incisional hernias include: correction of pre-operative risk factors (malnutrition), optimising respiratory status, correcting jaundice and uraemia, weight loss and meticulous surgical technique. Prophylactic antibiotics should be administered per-operatively where contamination has occurred. Wound closure should be with a non-absorbable monofilament (nylon, polypropylene). Suture bites should be 1 cm with a 1 cm spacing between successive sutures so that a suture to wound length ratio of 4:1 results.

5.4 Incisional hernias require operative repair and should be treated by either reconstruction using native tissues or placement of a non-absorbable mesh to bridge the defect.

5.5 This patient has a narrow-necked sac in which small bowel had become incarcerated and subsequently strangulated. A resection of all infarcted bowel is necessary.

Case 6 – Parastomal hernia/prolapse

6.1 Parastomal hernia.

6.2 The incidence of parastomal hernias ranges from 10% for paraileostomal hernias, up to 50% for paracolostomy hernias.

6.3 Paraileostomal hernias result in pain or discomfort. Paracolostomy hernias are usually larger in size, are bulky, cosmetically unappealing, and lead to seepage.

6.4 The majority of patients are asymptomatic and only 15% require repair. Surgical options include:

1 local repair (musculoaponeurotic repair, prosthetic mesh repair);

2 translocation of stoma with closure of the original defect.

6.5 Stomal prolapse.

Case 7 – Lipoma

7.1   Lipoma – this is the most common subcutaneous swelling.

7.2   Lipomas are benign lesions composed of adult-type fat cells and are usually enclosed within a fibrous capsule. The risk of malignant change is negligible. There are a few cases reporting sarcomatous change in large long-standing lipomas.

7.3   The only regions where lipomas are not found are the scalp, palm or sole since fatty tissue here is held within fibrous septae. They are most commonly seen around the head and neck, abdominal wall and thigh.

7.4   An encapsulated lipoma is being shelled from the surrounding tissue.

7.5   Dercum's disease.

Case 8 – Squamous cell carcinoma

8.1   There is an ulcerated lesion which has raised everted edges. This is the typical appearance of a squamous cell carcinoma.

8.2   Important predisposing factors include:

1   ultraviolet and ionising radiation exposure;

2   pre-malignant conditions – senile keratosis, Bowen's disease, lupus vulgaris, erythroplasia of Queyrat, Paget's disease;

3   inherited – xeroderma pigmentosum, albinism;

4   chronic irritation – Marjolin's ulcer, leukoplakia, varicose ulcers, arsenic, osteomyelitic sinuses, Kangri cancer of Kashmir, Kang cancer of China;

5   infection – human papilloma types 5 and 8.

8.3   Comparable results may be obtained by treatment with either radiotherapy or surgery. Tumours spread via lymphatics and if there is evidence of nodal disease at presentation, a nodal dissection should be performed.

8.4   Eighty per cent will be cured by either radiotherapy or surgery. Patients previously treated with radiotherapy who develop recurrences can be treated by surgical excision and patients undergoing excision of the primary may subsequently be treated with either surgery or radiotherapy.

8.5   Marjolin's ulcer.

Case 9 – Basal cell carcinoma

9.1 There is an area of central ulceration surrounded by a raised, rolled, pearly edge. This is typical of a basal cell carcinoma (rodent ulcer).

9.2 The most important aetiological factors are ultraviolet light exposure and fair skin.

9.3 Lesions are classically seen on the face above the line joining the angle of the mouth and the ear lobe.

9.4 Basal carcinomas may be treated by wide local excision (with a 1 cm margin) with or without skin grafting or by radiotherapy. In both instances the cure rate is around 90%.

9.5 This is a pigmented basal cell carcinoma. The important differential diagnosis is a malignant melanoma.

Case 10 – Melanoma

10.1 The lesion has an irregular edge, an irregular surface and shows variegated colouration. The diagnosis is malignant melanoma. Other stigmata of melanoma include recent increase in size, bleeding, ulceration, satellite lesions and pain.

10.2 The primary treatment of such a lesion is local excision with a minimum of 1 cm margin.

10.3 The main factor influencing prognosis is the histopathologic stage of the melanoma. This may be reported either as a Breslow thickness or as a Clark level. The Breslow thickness measures depth of invasion in millimeters whilst the Clark depth is an anatomical measurement. Other prognostic factors relate to the location of the primary tumour and the growth pattern of the tumour (superficial, nodular).

10.4 This patient has evidence of metastatic malignant melanoma with numerous in-transit lesions on the anterior aspect of the upper leg. Treatment options include:

1 surgery – excision of recurrent disease;

2 radiotherapy – large dose fractions;

3 chemotherapy – systemic or localised using limb perfusion;

4 immunotherapy – interleukin 2.

10.5 This is a Hutchinson's freckle or lentigo maligna. The mean age at diagnosis is 70 years, they are found on sun-exposed areas and occur most commonly in females. They represent around 10% of melanomas and have a better prognosis than other melanomas.

Case 11 – Subungual melanoma

11.1 The differential diagnosis includes melanoma, pigmented naevus and subungual haematoma.

11.2 The diagnosis should be established by performing a wide excisional biopsy. The diagnosis of this lesion was melanoma.

11.3 Melanomas are also found on the mucous membranes of the nose, mouth, anal canal, uveal tract and intestine.

11.4 The draining lymph nodes should be fully examined as should the abdomen for a palpable liver edge.

11.5 A subungual melanoma should be treated by amputation of the digit at the metacarpo/metatarsophalangeal joint.

Case 12 – Keratoacanthoma

12.1 There is a well-circumscribed lesion which has an irregular surface with smooth sides and central umbilication. There is also a variation in colour with a dark and crusty central core.

12.2 The appearances are typical of a keratoacanthoma (molluscum sebaceum), a lesion which is believed to arise from hyperplasia of hair follicle epithelia and metaplasia of sebaceous glands. They usually occur in the elderly in areas exposed to sunlight. The central plug consists of keratin and may bleed if disturbed.

12.3 Basal cell carcinoma, squamous cell carcinoma and melanoma must be included in any differential.

12.4 Lesions gradually regress over a period of 6–12 months without any treatment, leaving an irregular depressed scar. If there is any doubt as to the diagnosis they may be excised with adequate margins and sent for histological examination.

12.5 No.

Case 13 – Ingrowing toenail/onychogryphosis

13.1 There is marked inflammation with granulation tissue evident and proximal cellulitis. The diagnosis is ingrowing toenail (onychocryptosis).

13.2 The condition may occur at any age but is most commonly seen in children and young adults. The underlying cause is pressure necrosis of the nail wall due to persistent contact with the nail bed.

13.3 A Zadik's operation should be performed. The important steps are insertion of a local anaesthetic ring block of the digital nerves (n.b. No adrenaline*). The nail is removed and the germinal matrix of the nail bed is either excised completely or treated with phenol.

13.4 The diagnosis is onychogryphosis. The condition occurs when over-proliferation of the germinal matrix cells leads to excessive growth of the nail plate.

13.5 Patients should undergo regular manicure to prevent trauma to adjacent toes and secondary infections. Definitive treatment is a Zadik's procedure.

*Adrenaline should always be avoided when performing surgery on the fingers, nose, toes and penis.

Case 14 – Sebaceous cyst

14.1 Sebaceous cyst. They are true cysts lined by keratinising squamous epithelium resulting from obstruction of the mouth of a sebaceous gland and accumulation of keratinous debris.

14.2 They may occur in any region in which sebaceous glands are found (i.e. anywhere except palms and soles). Common sites include the face, ear lobe, back, scrotum and vulva.

14.3 Sebaceous cysts are soft and smooth, elicit fluctuance and are adherent to underlying fascia. They are usually seen to have a characteristic punctum.

14.4 An eliptical skin incision is made encompassing the punctum. The cyst is freed up by blunt dissection, taking care not to puncture the contents, and is removed.

14.5 Sebaceous horn. Other complications include infection, calcification, ulceration (Cock's peculiar tumour) and occasionally malignant transformation. The presence of multiple cysts may alert to the presence of Gardiner's syndrome in which intestinal polyposis, desmoid tumours and osteomas are also seen.

Case 15 – Ganglion

15.1 A ganglion.

15.2 A young adult presenting with a tense, painless swelling on the dorsum of the wrist.

15.3 Other common sites include the dorsum of the foot, flexor aspect of the fingers and over the peroneal tendons.

15.4 Proposed aetiologies include a benign tumour of the joint capsule/tendon sheath or a degenerative process of the tendon sheath/joint capsule secondary to trauma.

15.5 Under local anaesthetic, the ganglion is carefully mobilised from surrounding tissue taking care not to puncture its wall. Despite good technique, however, one-third will recur.

Case 16 – Hidradenitis suppurativa

16.1 Hidradenitis suppurativa.

16.2 The initial pathology is occlusion of the ducts of the apocrine glands by antigen–antibody complexes. This predisposes to chronic infection and abscess formation by organisms such as staphylococci, streptococci and anaerobes.

16.3 The axillae, perianal, submammary and inguinal regions.

16.4 Early presentations may be managed non-operatively with antibiotic therapy (e.g. metronidazole). Extensive disease requires surgical excision of all affected skin with either primary closure, skin grafting or healing by secondary intention depending on the body site affected.

16.5 Despite radical surgery there is a significant recurrence rate that is lower for perianal and axillary disease (<5%) and greatest for inguinal/perineal/submammary (up to 50%).

Case 17 – Pyogenic granuloma

17.1 There is a 1 cm smooth bright red pedunculated lesion with evidence of recent bleeding.

17.2 Pyogenic granuloma.

17.3 The condition is most commonly seen in children and young adults (hands and faces) and is also common in pregnant women (lips and gums).

17.4 No. The lesion was originally believed to be a granulation reaction to infection – hence the name. The lesion is in fact a benign rapidly growing capillary haemangioma.

17.5 The lesion should be curetted with diathermy to its base.

Case 18 – Von Recklinghausen's disease

18.1 The diagnosis is multiple neurofibromatosis. There are two forms of the disease:

type I – bilateral acoustic neuromas but skin lesions may be sparse;

type II – more benign outlook (von Recklinghausen's disease). The other characteristic dermatological lesions are: *café au lait* spots (80% have more than six patches); multiple freckles over the axillae, lower abdomen, buttocks and thighs; and areas of depigmentation.

18.2 Von Recklinghausen's disease may present as a plexiform mass (bag of worms), thickened peripheral nerves, or deafness due to a neurofibroma affecting the 8th cranial nerve.

18.3 There is an association between neurofibromas and medullary carcinoma of thyroid/phaeochromocytoma as part of the multiple endocrine neoplasia IIb syndrome. There is also a higher incidence of gliomas and meningiomas in patients with neurofibromas.

18.4 The disease is autosomally dominantly inherited with variable gene expression.

18.5 Treatment is generally on a symptomatic basis as patients often have many neurofibromas. There is an argument for excision of lesions affecting major nerves. Malignant degeneration may occur in up to 10%.

Case 19 – Rectus sheath haematoma

19.1 The differential includes appendix mass, caecal carcinoma, Crohn's disease and diverticular disease.

19.2 There is a large haematoma limited to the rectus sheath.

19.3 Haematomas may occur spontaneously, following minor trauma such as sneezing/coughing or following strenuous exercise. They are also seen in patients with connective tissue disorders, in patients on anticoagulant therapy and in individuals with haematological disorders.

19.4 The underlying disorder is believed to be poor elasticity in the inferior epigastric vessels.

19.5 The patient should be managed non-operatively with correction of hypovolaemia, anaemia and clotting abnormalities. Surgery is reserved for those patients in whom conservative management fails.

Case 20 – Wound infection

20.1 There is evidence of a deep wound infection. Infection is the most common complication of surgery with an incidence varying from 1% for clean operations (e.g. hernia) to 25% for contaminated procedures (e.g. colonic operations).

20.2 Predisposing factors include: pre-operative skin infections; contamination from a perforated viscus; malnutrition (hypoproteinaemia, hypovitaminosis); diabetes mellitus; malignancy; corticosteroids; airborne infection in theatre; haematoma formation; contaminated operations; nasal carriage of organisms by patients and staff (e.g. staphylococci).

20.3 Organisms commonly isolated are staphylococci, coliforms (*E. coli, Proteus, Pseudomonas*), anaerobes and haemolytic streptococci.

20.4 The patient should be treated with broad spectrum intravenous antibiotics. The wound should be reviewed regularly and any abscess or necrotic tissue treated.

20.5 If neglected there may be total breakdown and wound dehiscence. This is characterised by the 'pink fluid sign' – discharge of a blood-tinged serosanguinous fluid 2 days before wound breakdown.

Upper gastrointestinal

Case 21 – Adenocarcinoma of the oesophagus

21.1 Barium swallow showing a stricture in the lower oesophagus (Figure 21a) and an endoscopic ultra-sound showing a T3 N1 adenocarcinoma of the oesophagus (Figure 21b).

21.2 T1 = Tumour invades mucosa or submucosa

T2 = Tumour invades muscularis propria

T3 = Tumour invades adventitia

T4 = Tumour invades neighbouring structures

N0 = No evidence of regional lymph node metastasis

N1 = Evidence of regional lymph node metastasis

M0 = No evidence of distant metastasis

M1 = Evidence of distant metastasis

21.3 The appropriate treatment is oesophagectomy. The choice of surgical approach depends upon the tumour location and the surgeon's prefer-ence. They are:

1 Ivor Lewis procedure (right fifth interspace thoracotomy and upper midline laparotomy) which is used for mid- and lower-third tumours;

2 left thoraco-abdominal approach (oblique left upper quadrant laparotomy continued through the left sixth rib space) which is best for lower third and cardia tumours;

3 trans-hiatal approach (upper midline laparo-tomy and cervical incision) which avoids a tho-racotomy.

21.4 The most common complications following oesophagectomy are respiratory problems (atelec-tasis, pneumonia) occurring in up to 50%. Anastomotic leak is the most feared of complica-tions (5%) as an intrathoracic anastomotic leak has a high mortality. Other complications are atrial fibrillation and the development of an anastomotic stricture.

21.5 The post-operative mortality is in the order of 5–10% and the 5 year survival following surgery approximately 20%.

Case 22 – Squamous cell carcinoma of the oesophagus

22.1 A barium swallow showing a filling defect in the middle third of the oesophagus (Figure 22a) and an endoscopic view (Figure 22b) showing a squamous cell carcinoma.

22.2 The incidence ranges from 5 per 100 000 population for most parts of Western Europe and North America to more than 100 per 100 000 population for the Linxian region of China and the Caspian region of Iran. Other areas with a high incidence are Brittany, France and the Transkei, South Africa. The condition affects principally males (M:F 5:1) between the ages of 50–70 years. In the US black males are affected three times more commonly than white males.

22.3 The gentleman has evidence of distant metastases (supraclavicular lymphadenopathy) making curative surgical resection unfeasible. In addition, he has evidence of chronic obstructive airways disease with significantly compromised pulmonary function. Both of these factors would independently mitigate against undertaking curative oesophagectomy; he is thus only amenable to palliative treatment. Other contra-indications to curative resection are a history of myocardial infarction within the last 6 months, uncontrolled angina, a predicted left ventricular ejection fraction <40%, hepatic cirrhosis and chronic renal failure. Although physiological status is the primary consideration age >75 years is generally considered to be a contra-indication to oesophagectomy.

22.4 Appropriate treatments would include oesophageal intubation, with either a plastic endoprosthesis or a covered metal stent, laser therapy or external beam radiotherapy.

22.5 Risk factors for the development of squamous cell carcinoma are heavy consumption of alcohol, cigarette smoking, molybdenum deficiency (putative cause in China), achalasia, corrosive strictures, tylosis type A, Paterson–Brown–Kelly syndrome (post-cricoid web) and scleroderma. Tobacco and alcohol act synergistically as risk factors.

Case 23 – Gastro-oesophageal reflux disease

23.1 The photographs show the endoscopic appearance of grade 2 oesophagitis (Figure 23a) and Barrett's oesophagus (grade 4 oesophagitis) (Figure 23b).

23.2 The Savary-Miller grading system.

Grade 1: Erythema at the squamo-columnar junction

Grade 2: Non-confluent linear ulceration in the lower 5 cm of the oesophagus

Grade 3: Confluent linear ulceration in the lower 5 cm of the oesophagus

Grade 4: Circumferential fibrosis, stricture, Barrett's oesophagus (intestinal metaplasia)

23.3 Treatment is initially medical with a proton-pump inhibitor, such as omeprazole at a dose of 20 mg twice daily. The sinister complication is the development of adenocarcinoma of the oesophagus. The relative risk for the development of adenocarcinoma of the oesophagus in patients with Barrett's oesophagus is in the order of 50–100.

23.4 Oesophageal manometry and ambulatory 24 hour oesophageal pH studies. These would be used to determine the competence of the lower oesophageal sphincter and a quantification of the amount of oesophageal acid exposure (normal total percentage time spent below pH 4.0 is <4.4%).

23.5 Surgery. The operative treatment (anti-reflux surgery) of gastro-oesophageal reflux disease is by a fundoplication, the most commonly employed being a Nissen fundoplication. Formerly performed through an upper midline laparotomy, the procedure is now performed laparoscopically. Some surgeons advocate a tailored approach, that is performing a 360 degree wrap on patients with normal distal oesophageal motility and a 270 degree wrap on patients with poor distal oesophageal motility.

Case 24 – Achalasia

24.1 Figure 24a is a barium swallow showing the characteristic features of achalasia, a dilated oesophagus above a narrowed oesophago-gastric junction ('bird's beak deformity'). Figure 24b is the appearance of wet swallows obtained during stationary oesophageal manometry and Figure 24c is a vector–volume manometry tracing of the lower oesophageal sphincter.

24.2 The characteristic manometric features of achalasia are:

1 absence of peristaltic waves in the oesophagus;

2 a high resting intra-oesophageal pressure;

3 impaired lower oesophageal sphincter relaxation;

4 high resting lower oesophageal sphincter pressure. Not uncommonly the resting intra-oesophageal pressure rises during the manometric evaluation as a result of distension of the oesophagus by the infused water.

24.3 The incidence of the condition is approximately 5 per million per year in the UK. It occurs worldwide and affects both genders equally. The peak incidence is between the ages of 30–60 years.

24.4 Endoscopy may be normal. Possible findings are a dilated oesophagus, absent peristalsis, food residue or a tight lower oesophageal sphincter.

24.5 Conservative therapy with oral nitrates or calcium channel antagonists may provide some temporary symptomatic relief, but is unlikely to result in permanent symptom control. Further management of this condition is directed towards controlled disruption of the lower oesophageal sphincter. This can be achieved endoscopically by balloon dilatation or operatively (open or thoracoscopic) by oesophagomyotomy. Complications of treatment are oesophageal perforation and gastro-oesophageal reflux disease.

Case 25 – Complicated peptic ulcer disease

25.1 The chest radiograph (Figure 25a) shows free gas under the left hemi-diaphragm indicating the presence of air within the peritoneal cavity. Figure 25b is a per-operative photograph showing a perforated duodenal ulcer.

25.2 Typically perforated duodenal ulcers produce acute-onset epigastric pain followed by the development of more generalised abdominal pain. Sometimes right iliac fossa pain occurs as a result of duodenogastric contents accumulating at this site under gravity. Nausea is common, but vomiting *per se* is uncommon. Examination of the abdomen may reveal distention and a 'boardlike' character on palpation due to involuntary contraction of the rectus abdominis muscles. Auscultation reveals either a paucity or absence of bowel sounds. Systemic signs include fever, tachycardia, tachypnoea and a dry tongue.

25.3 Some surgeons advocate a conservative approach to the management of perforated duodenal ulcer – intravenous fluids, antibacterials and passage of a nasogastric tube. In this instance the patient must be closely monitored with surgical intervention if any signs of clinical deterioration occur. Most would advocate laparotomy however and oversewing of the ulcer, with many placing a small patch of omentum over the ulcer site. Some surgeons would combine this with a definitive procedure such as truncal vagotomy or highly selective vagotomy. In some patients, those with uncontrolled haemorrhage or large perforations not amenable to primary closure, more radical resectional surgery is required.

25.4 The other complications of duodenal ulcer disease are obstruction, fistulation and haemorrhage.

25.5 Duodenal ulcers typically affect young males below the age of 50 years. Predisposing factors include cigarette smoking; alcohol; the use of corticosteroids, aspirin and non-steroidal anti-inflammatory agents.

Case 26 – Adenocarcinoma of the stomach

26.1 Gastric carcinoma.

26.2 There is wide variation in the incidence of gastric carcinoma, with a high incidence seen in parts of Asia (Japan, China) and South America (Chile, Costa Rica, Columbia). In Europe the countries with a high incidence of the disease are Russia, Portugal, Italy and Poland. Worldwide males are affected twice as commonly as females. The peak incidence is between the ages of 50–70 years.

26.3 There has been a shift towards a more proximal tumour location, such that carcinoma of the gastric cardia is the most common tumour location. There has been a trebling in the incidence of carcinoma of the gastric cardia and adenocarcinoma of the lower oesophagus in the UK over the last decade. These two conditions share similar epidemiological features and probably arise by a similar mechanism. The incidence of carcinoma of the gastric antrum and body has remained unchanged in the UK.

26.4 Much of the work on disease aetiology relates to carcinoma of the gastric body and antrum in high risk areas such as Japan. There is some evidence of familial clustering of the condition suggesting a genetic predisposition in a small percentage of index patients. Putative risk factors include the following dietary factors: high salt diet, high intake of starch, ingestion of smoked and pickled foods. In contrast protective dietary factors are the consumption of fresh fruit and vegetables, milk and use of refrigeration. Cigarette smokers and individuals of blood group A have a greater relative risk. Risk factors for the development of carcinoma of the cardia are less well studied but include an association with high body mass index, a high dietary consumption of fat, cigarette smoking and high alcohol intake. Premalignant gastric disorders include pernicious anaemia, chronic atrophic gastritis, Ménétrier's disease, adenomatous polyps, juvenile polyps and prior gastric resection.

26.5 The treatment depends upon the disease stage at presentation. Palliation is appropriate for patients with distant metastases or those unfit for surgical resection. Palliative options include no surgery, a palliative resection or a bypass procedure. Curative surgery comprises gastrectomy. The extent of resection is still the subject of debate. Retrospective data from Japan and Germany have suggested a survival advantage for D2 radical gastrectomy. However, preliminary data from two prospective randomised controlled trials from the UK and the Netherlands have failed to show a survival advantage for the D2 radical gastrectomy over the conventional D1 gastrectomy. The latter is probably the most commonly employed operation in the UK.

Case 27 – Stromal tumour of the stomach

27.1 Figure 27a is a barium meal and Figure 27b is a resection specimen showing a pedunculated tumour of the mid gastric body along the greater curve. The most likely diagnosis is a gastrointestinal stromal tumour, formerly known as leiomyoma or leiomyosarcoma.

27.2 The differential diagnosis includes carcinoma, lymphoma, adenomatous polyp and schwannoma.

27.3 The peak incidence is between the ages of 50–70 years with males and females being equally affected. The stomach is the most common site for gastrointestinal stromal tumours.

27.4 Gastric stromal tumours are a common finding at autopsy but only a small proportion of these are symptomatic ante-mortem. The most common presenting features are those of upper gastrointestinal haemorrhage (up to 90%) with haematemesis, melaena and anaemia. Other features include epigastric pain, weight loss and the presence of a palpable mass. Stromal tumours may be incidental findings at the time of laparotomy or gastroscopy for unrelated reasons.

27.5 Treatment is surgical excision with a 2 cm margin of surrounding tissue. The biological behaviour of gastrointestinal stromal tumours is difficult to predict. In general the larger the lesion the greater the number of mitoses, and the greater the degree of cellular atypia the more malignant is its biological behaviour.

Case 28 – Oesophageal varices

28.1 Figure 28a shows spider naevi over the anterior chest wall, Figure 28b shows gynaecomastia and hepatosplenomegaly. Figure 28c is an endoscopic photograph of oesophageal varices. All are features of hepatic cirrhosis.

28.2 The underlying pathophysiology is that of portal hypertension. In the distal oesophagus venous communications between the portal (left gastric vein) and systemic (azygous vein) circulation dilate to form varices that run in submucosal columns (numbering between 3–5) in the oesophagus. The precise trigger for variceal rupture is unclear – suggested mechanisms include reflux of gastric acid resulting in erosion of mucosa overlying the varix and when the variceal pressure reaches a critical value. Haemorrhage from oesophageal varices is the most serious complication of portal hypertension, being responsible for around one-third of deaths in cirrhotic patients.

28.3 Emergency treatment of ruptured oesophageal varices is appropriate resuscitation of the patient, endoscopic sclerotherapy and balloon tamponade with a Sengstaken–Blakemore tube. The Sengstaken tube is deflated at 24 hours and if bleeding has stopped is removed 48 hours after insertion. If bleeding is not controlled repeat sclerotherapy is undertaken and the tube left inflated for a further 24 hours after an interval of 1 hour deflation. Emergency surgery is indicated for failed medical therapy. Any coagulation defect should be corrected with fresh frozen plasma. Appropriate sclerosant agents include sodium tetradecyl sulphate, ethanolamine oleate and ethanol. The former is the most widely used in the UK. 1–2 mL are injected either into the varix directly or into the para-variceal tissue.

28.4 Complications of injection sclerotherapy are oesophageal ulceration at the injection sites and oesophageal perforation. Complications of balloon tamponade are ischaemic necrosis of the oesophageal mucosa, oesophageal perforation and aspiration pneumonitis.

28.5 Alteration of the underlying portal hypertension may be achieved surgically by the creation of a shunt between the portal and the systemic circulation or radiologically by transjugular intrahepatic porta-systemic shunting (TIPS).

Case 29 – Uncomplicated peptic ulcer disease

29.1 Gastric ulcer.

29.2 *Helicobacter pylori*. Identification of *Helicobacter pylori* can be achieved in a number of ways: urease test, histology (Giemsa stain), breath test and serology. The first two are the most commonly used methods.

29.3 Treatment is by *Helicobacter* eradication therapy. This comprises triple therapy (two antibacterials and a proton-pump inhibitor such as omeprazole in a dose of 20 mg bd). Antibacterials commonly used are amoxycillin, clarithromycin, erythromycin and metronidazole. Antibacterial therapy is for 1 week and acid suppression therapy for 4–6 weeks.

29.4 Patients with gastric ulcers should be followed up by repeat gastroscopy to confirm the occurrence of ulcer healing. The ulcer margins should be biopsied to exclude malignancy.

29.5 Gastric ulcers occur predominantly in patients over the age of 50, with females being affected more commonly. As with duodenal ulcer disease predisposing factors include cigarette smoking; alcohol; the use of corticosteroids, aspirin and non-steroidal anti-inflammatory agents.

Case 30 – Benign oesophageal stricture

30.1 A benign oesophageal stricture.

30.2 The aetiology of this condition is gastro-oesophageal reflux disease. Repetitive injury from gastric contents ultimately results in chronic inflammation, ulceration and circumferential fibrosis of the oesophagus. Patients with strictures have more severe reflux disease than those without strictures; in general, they reflux in the supine posture as well as in the upright posture.

30.3 Other causes of oesophageal stricturing are anastomotic, radiotherapy, corrosive ingestion, drug-induced (non-steroidal anti-inflammatory agents, potassium chloride) and infective causes (immunosuppressed patients).

30.4 The majority of these patients are elderly. Most present with a history of dysphagia. There may or may not be a long history of reflux symptoms (heartburn, regurgitation).

30.5 Most strictures can be managed medically with a combination of acid suppression (proton-pump inhibitors) and oesophageal dilatation endoscopically. These measures, however, do nothing to alter the underlying pathophysiology. Thus physiologically fit patients should undergo an anti-reflux procedure such as a fundoplication. If there has been significant oesophageal shortening, an oesophageal lengthening procedure, such as a Collis gastroplasty, will be necessary.

Case 31 – Subphrenic abscess

31.1 A chest radiograph showing air-fluid levels below both hemi-diaphragms indicating bilateral subphrenic abscesses. The subphrenic spaces are the most common site for the development of intra-abdominal abscesses. In septic surgical patients in whom pulmonary and pelvic sepsis has been excluded it is important to consider subphrenic abscess as a possibility ('...pus somewhere, pus nowhere, pus under the diaphragm').

31.2 Aetiologies include spontaneous abdominal organ perforation (peptic ulcer disease, diverticular disease, Crohn's disease, appendicitis, cholecystitis, intestinal infarction), penetrating injuries, and following abdominal surgery (open and laparoscopic).

31.3 The microbiology of subphrenic abscesses is polymicrobial, usually Gram-negatives and anaerobes.

31.4 Plain radiography may show the following findings: air-fluid levels, pleural effusion or hemi-diaphragm elevation. Confirmation of the diagnosis is generally by either ultrasound scanning or computerised tomography. The former is the most widely used, avoids ionising radiation, is portable and thus more easily performed on a ventilated patient on the intensive care unit.

31.5 Treatment is by drainage and appropriate antibacterial therapy. Drainage can usually be performed percutaneously under imaging guidance. Surgical drainage (transabdominal approach) is employed in those patients that have failed to respond to percutaneous drainage or in those abscesses not amenable to percutaneous drainage.

Hepatobiliary and pancreas

Case 32 – Cholangiocarcinoma

32.1 The history suggests obstructive jaundice and the differential lies between: common duct stones, iatrogenic strictures, inflammatory stricture secondary to chronic pancreatitis, hilar compression from malignant adenopathy and primary neoplasms (pancreatic, duodenal, gallbladder, common bile duct – cholangiocarcinoma, hilar – Klatskin tumour).

32.2 The ultrasound demonstrates dilatation of the proximal common bile duct and the intrahepatic bile ducts.

32.3 This is a CT scan demonstrating intra- and extra-hepatic bile duct dilatation. There is no evidence of a mass either in the pancreatic head or at the porta hepatis.

32.4 This is a percutaneous transhepatic cholangiogram demonstrating intra- and extra-hepatic duct dilatation with obstruction of the mid common bile duct level. In the absence of previous surgery this appearance is suggestive of a cholangiocarcinoma. A plastic stent has been placed across the obstruction into the duodenum allowing bile drainage and relief from the jaundice.

32.5 An expandable metal stent could be placed endoscopically. These are reported to have a longer patency, with less stent migration, less tumour overgrowth and fewer infection episodes than plastic stents. Operative options include tumour bypass with a loop of jejunum anastomosed to the proximal bile duct or segment III duct. In early tumours in young, fit patients a Whipple's procedure may offer a cure. The overall 5 year survival is close to 0% but for patients undergoing curative resections it is around 25%.

Case 33 – Hydatid disease

33.1 The likely diagnosis is hydatid disease of the liver, the causative organism being *Echinococcus granulosus*. Serological tests to identify the parasite include complement fixation, indirect fluorescent antibody testing, enzyme-linked immunosorbent assays and a specific immunoelectrophoretogram, the latter being the most specific.

33.2 The CT demonstrates a cystic lesion in the right lobe. The large (mother) cyst contains several smaller daughter cysts. In addition to showing the characteristic appearances of hydatid, the scan also gives information on the extent of the disease and the anatomical relationships of the cyst.

33.3 Options are non-operative and operative. Drug treatment of hydatid is with albendazole or mebendazole. Surgical options include marsupialisation of the cyst, evacuation and drainage of the cyst or resection of cyst and a rim of surrounding tissue if the cyst is peripheral.

33.4 Good exposure is required through a generous incision. The area around the cyst is packed with sponges soaked in 3% saline solution. The cyst contents are aspirated and hypertonic saline is instilled into the cyst taking care not to spill the cyst contents. The cyst is then drained and a careful inspection made for residual daughter cysts. The laminated membrane of the cyst is then excised. A careful inspection is then made for biliary leakage prior to closure.

33.5 The cumulative recurrence following surgery is around 22% with disease manifesting usually within 3 years.

Case 34 – Primary liver cancer

34.1 The ultrasound demonstrates a large solid mass within the left lobe of the liver.

34.2 The CT demonstrates a tumour in the left lobe of the liver. It has an irregular outline and there is evidence of central necrosis. The image has been enhanced by the use of the contrast agent lipiodol which localises in the tumour. The appearances are consistent with a primary liver cancer.

34.3 The most common pathology is hepatocellular carcinoma (HCC) which may be the most common visceral neoplasm world-wide. Cholangiocarcinomas arise from the biliary epithelium and are the second most common primary malignancy. Angiosarcomas are rare but highly malignant. In a child the differential would also include hepatoblastoma.

34.4 The predisposing factors for hepatocellular carcinoma are hepatitis B and C infection, alcohol consumption, blood group B, hepatic adenoma, porphyria cutanea tarda, haemochromatosis, aflatoxin intake, plant alkaloids, androgens, vinyl chloride, thorium dioxide, smoking and organo-chloride pesticides. The fibrolamellar variant of HCC is associated with androgen abuse. Cholangiocarcinomas are associated with chronic cholestasis, cirrhosis, haemochromatosis, ulcerative colitis, choledochal cysts and infection with *Clonorchis sinensis*. Important risk factors for angiosarcoma are exposure to vinylchloride monomer, thorium dioxide, arsenic and anabolic steroids.

34.5 Surgical resection is the treatment of choice for HCC though the resectability rate is low. Resection may be performed on an anatomical basis or by wedge excision which is advantageous in patients with cirrhosis. The results of transplantation for HCC are poor with the exception of the fibrolamellar variant. The response rate for chemotherapy is disappointingly low. The overall outlook is usually hopeless although patients with small resectable tumours in non-cirrhotic livers have a 5 year survival of around up to 30%. The fibrolamellar HCC has a better outlook with a median survival of 3–5 years.

Case 35 – Gallstones

35.1 The radiograph demonstrates gallbladder calculi which are only evident in 10% of cases. The likely diagnosis is biliary colic.

35.2 The ultrasound demonstrates multiple hyperechoic calculi within the gallbladder which cast acoustic shadows. This appearance is typical of gallstones.

35.3 The prevalence of gallstones from cadaveric studies is approximately 1 in 10 of the population; however, only 20% will experience symptoms.

35.4 The majority of stones (80%) are a mixture of cholesterol, bilirubin and calcium (smooth or faceted, light brown and laminated), a small number are cholesterol stones (large, yellow) and some are pigment stones (small, black). The pathogenesis of gallstones is related to abnormalities in the relative concentrations of cholesterol, lecithin and bile salts. Risk factors include *Salmonella typhi* infection, foreign bodies, lipid abnormalities, Crohn's disease, ileal resection, oral contraceptive pill and liver disease. Pigment stones are associated with haemolytic anaemia, cirrhosis, *Escherichia coli* and *Ascaris lumbricoides*.

35.5 Figure 35c demonstrates a gallstone ileus with the gallstone visible on the right margin of the film and Figure 35d is an operative picture showing the gallstone in the ileum, close to erosion through the wall. Other complications of gallstones include: acute cholecystitis, chronic cholecystitis, pancreatitis, cholangitis, empyema, mucocoele and perforation of the gallbladder.

Case 36 – Common bile duct stone

36.1 The differential is between an iatrogenic bile duct injury and a retained common bile duct (CBD) stone. CBD stones are found in up to 15% of patients undergoing cholecystectomy.

36.2 Figure 36a shows an endoscopic retrograde cholangiopancreaticogram (ERCP) which confirms the presence of stones in the duct. In Figure 36b a sphincterotome is being passed in order to perform a sphincterotomy.

36.3 Figure 36c shows a Dormia basket retrieving a stone and Figure 36d illustrates decompression of the biliary system with a stent prior to operative removal of an impacted stone.

36.4 The morbidity of ERCP is <10% and mortality <1%. The main complications of ERCP include cholangitis, haemorrhage, pancreatitis and perforation which may be intra- or retro-peritoneal.

36.5 Other options for dealing with common duct stones include: open exploration of the CBD; open or laparoscopic choledochoscopy and stone extraction; dissolution therapy; lithotripsy.

Case 37 – Air in biliary tree

37.1 The plain abdominal film demonstrates air within the biliary tree. The differential diagnosis includes ascending cholangitis, post operation (biliary-enteric anastamosis), post ERCP and gallstone ileus.

37.2 Charcot's triad consists of the symptoms of right upper quadrant pain, jaundice and fever, features characteristic of cholangitis.

37.3 The ultrasound demonstrates a thickened and distended gallbladder consistent with an empyema.

37.4 The CT confirms the presence of an empyema of the gallbladder and also demonstrates multiple liver abscesses.

37.5 There is a significant mortality (10%) due to septic shock and liver failure. It is important to fully resuscitate patients and administer broad spectrum antibiotics. In the case of an identifiable source for sepsis, and the presence of multiple abscesses an operative approach with cholecystectomy and drainage of the abscess cavities is recommended. If there is a single abscess percutaneous drainage may be performed.

Case 38 – Laparoscopic cholecystectomy

38.1 A pneumoperitoeum is being established. The first step is to deflate the bladder and stomach by inserting a urinary catheter and nasogastric tube and then to position the patient in a Trendelenberg position. The needle is inserted perpendicular to the abdominal wall and its position is checked (free movement, drop test, saline injection/aspiration, percussion). A pressure of about 12 mm Hg is maintained and insufflation continued until 3.5–4 litres of carbon dioxide are present within the peritoneal cavity.

38.2 A trocar is being inserted using a closed technique in Figure 38b and using an open (Hassan) technique in Figure 38c. The open method does not require an introducer and has a lesser incidence of visceral injury.

38.3 Calot's triangle is a triangular space bounded by the liver, common hepatic duct and the cystic duct. The cystic artery and node are found within it.

38.4 Figure 38d is an intraoperative cholangiogram. The exact role of cholangiography in laparoscopic cholecystectomy is controversial with some authors recommending routine use and others not. The overall consensus is to perform cholangiography if clinical criteria are suggestive of CBD abnormalities or if the anatomy is unclear.

38.5 Complications are divided into laparoscopic and operation-related. The former include: abdominal wall bruising, subcutaneous emphysema, wound infection, visceral and vascular damage, haemorrhage, shoulder tip pain, subphrenic abscess and diathermy injuries. Complications specific to laparoscopic cholecystectomy include bile leak, bile duct division, iatrogenic strictures, hepatic ischaemia, gallstone fistula.

Case 39 – Bile duct injury

39.1 The likely diagnosis is an iatrogenic bile duct injury. The overall incidence of bile duct injuries following laparoscopic cholecystectomy in large series is between 0.3% and 0.5% compared with 0.2% for the open operation.

39.2 This ERCP demonstrates an abrupt occlusion to the common bile duct with no delineation of the intrahepatic biliary radicals. A clip is seen apparently occluding the bile duct.

39.3 The classic injury is misidentification of the common bile duct for the cystic duct. In this case the CBD is clipped and divided, the common hepatic duct is clipped and the intervening section of the biliary tree is resected. A second common mistake is division of the CBD distally and the cystic duct proximally leaving a biliary fistula. A tented CBD may also be mistaken for the cystic duct as may an aberrant right hepatic duct. Bile duct strictures present later and are usually related to diathermy injuries or malpositioning of clips. Both are related to ischaemic damage.

39.4 If the injury is recognised intraoperatively the operation can be converted to an open procedure. However, most are recognised during the post-operative course. In the case of bile duct transection, if there is adequate length, an anastomosis may be stented with a T-tube. The integrity of the anastomosis is checked with a cholangiogram prior to stent removal. If the duct is partially occluded a stent may be placed at the time of ERCP to maintain the luminal diameter during healing. For cases in which there is inadequate length of bile duct available, a choledochojejunostomy may be performed. In the case of more proximal injuries, a segment III biliary-enteric anastomosis may be performed. There are reports of a few cases of biliary injuries that have required liver transplantation.

39.5 This ERCP demonstrates a bile leak resulting in a collection in the gallbladder fossa. This complication is seen in approximately 1.5% of laparoscopic cholecystectomies. The most common causes are a displaced cystic duct clip and an unrecognised subvesical duct of Luschka, a slender biliary duct from the right lobe to the gallbladder. Other reasons include displacement of a clip from the cystic duct stump or laceration of a larger biliary duct.

Case 40 – Acute pancreatitis

40.1 The sign of periumbilical erythema and ecchymosis is Cullen's sign (indication of retroperitoneal haemorrhage – pancreatitis, ruptured ectopic pregnancy, leaking/rupture aneurysm). The probable diagnosis is acute pancreatitis. Hyperamylasaemia may also be seen in association with acute and chronic renal failure, salivary gland disease, liver disease, CBD stone, acute cholecystitis, peptic ulceration, Crohn's disease, mesenteric infarction, diabetic ketoacidosis and salpingitis.

40.2 Imrie's criteria are a series of prognostic indicators assessed within 24 hours of presentation and include age >55 years; WBC $>15 \times 10^9$, urea >6 mmol/L, glucose >10 mmol/L, calcium <2 mmol/L, albumin <32 g/L, O_2 <8 kPa and plasma lactate dehydrogenase >600 IU/L. A point is awarded for each variable and a score of 2 or more indicates a severe attack of pancreatitis. An alternative scoring system is Ransom's.

40.3 The two most common aetiological factors are gallstones and alcohol, each accounting for approximately 40% of cases. Other aetiological factors include ampullary obstruction, annular pancreas, pancreatic duct obstruction (cysts, calculi, tumours), hyperlipidaemia, hypercalcaemia, uraemia, trauma, post-ERCP, infection (mycoplasma, mumps, Coxsackie, *Clonorchis sinensis*), ischaemic, gynaecological (salpingitis, ruptured ectopic pregnancy), hypothermia, vascular (hypertension, SLE, PAN, cardiopulmonary bypass, leaking aortic aneurysm) and numerous drugs (azathioprine, oestrogens, thiazides).

40.4 The CT demonstrates a markedly oedematous pancreas with areas of early necrosis consistent with severe acute pancreatitis.

40.5 I: Careful monitoring – including urinary catheter, pulse oximetry, and central venous pressure monitoring if the pancreatitis is severe, in a high dependency unit. A nasogastric tube should also be passed to decompress the stomach.

II: Analgesia – usually require morphine although paradoxically this causes spasm of the sphincter of Oddi.

III: Fluid replacement – intravenous rehydration and avoidance of oral fluids. In severe pancreatitis dehydration leads to reduced splanchnic circulation and pancreatic ischaemia with subsequent necrosis.

IV: Oxygen therapy – to correct any hypoxaemia.

V: Regular re-assessment. If there is a deterioration a CT scan or MRI should be performed to look for necrosis. If there is a history of gallstones and ultrasound evidence of biliary obstruction, emergency ERCP and sphincterotomy should be performed. If there is a deterioration in respiratory function the patient should be moved to the intensive care unit and ventilated if necessary. In severe pancreatitis, total parenteral nutrition should be considered.

VI: Surgical interventions include peritoneal lavage to remove toxins, debridement of necrotic tissue and drainage of pancreatic abscesses.

Case 41 – Pancreatic pseudocyst

41.1 The CT demonstrates a large pseudocyst in the body of the pancreas. It is of homogenous density, has a well-defined wall, and is compressing the stomach anteriorly.

41.2 A pseudocyst results from leakage of enzyme-rich pancreatic juices from a severely inflamed pancreas. The wall of the pseudocyst consists of a combination of fibrous and granulation tissue and hence it is not a true cyst.

41.3 This CT demonstrates a stent *in situ* from the pseudocyst to the stomach following an endoscopic cyst-gastrostomy.

41.4 Pseudocysts can be drained to stomach, duodenum or small bowel and procedures can be carried out either endoscopically or surgically.

41.5 Systemic complications of acute pancreatitis: respiratory failure (21%), multiple organ failure (6%), renal failure (6%), cardiovascular collapse (4%) and disseminated intravascular coagulopathy (1%). Gastrointestinal: gastroparesis, jaundice and cholangitis may occur secondary to pancreatic oedema. Intra-abdominal: pancreatic ascites, pancreatic necrosis (4%), and pancreatic abscess (3%).

Case 42 – Chronic pancreatitis

42.1 This ERCP demonstrates a dilated main pancreatic duct ('chain of lakes' appearance) and duct ectasia of the secondary ducts, features typical of chronic pancreatitis.

42.2 Alcohol is the most common cause of chronic pancreatitis and accounts for around 70% of cases. Ductal obstruction due to post-traumatic stricturing, stones, pseudocysts, tumours or pancreas divisium leads to chronic obstructive pancreatitis. Other aetiologies include hypercalcaemia, malnutrition, cystic fibrosis and hereditary idiopathic chronic pancreatitis.

42.3 Pain is the most difficult aspect to manage and many patients require regular opiate analgesia. Patients are advised to stop drinking and to take regular small meals to reduce enzyme release. H2 blockers, in addition to treating associated duodenitis, also reduce pancreatic enzyme secretion. The somatostatin analogue octreotide also inhibits pancreatic function. If the pain persists a coeliac plexus block may be performed. Pancreatic exocrine function can be corrected with enzyme supplements which are taken regularly with food. The exact dose required depends on the degree of dysfunction and the size of the meal. If there is significant islet destruction the patient may develop diabetes mellitus which will require administration of insulin.

42.4 Surgical success depends on careful patient selection with particular reference to abstinence from alcohol consumption. Drainage procedures such as longitudinal pancreaticojejunostomy are employed when the pancreatic duct is dilated more than 8 mm. Resections of the pancreatic head, body or the whole gland depending on extent and location of disease.

42.5 At long-term follow-up following surgery 75% report freedom from pain, 15% are improved and the remainder are unchanged.

Case 43 – Adenocarcinoma pancreas

43.1 Courvoisier's law states that in the presence of painless jaundice, if the gallbladder is palpable then the cause is unlikely to be gallstones. The law is interpreted as: if in the presence of painless jaundice there is a palpable gallbladder the underlying cause is likely to be a carcinoma of the pancreas. This law holds true in approximately two-thirds of cases. Exceptions to this include infection with the liver fluke *Clonorchis sinensis* and gallstones impacted concurrently in the common bile duct and cystic duct.

43.2 There is a smooth tapering stricture at the lower end of the common bile duct where the tumour is encasing the duct and dilatation of both the common bile duct and the pancreatic duct (double duct sign). The ERCP allows cytology and brushings to be obtained and therefore establish a definite diagnosis.

43.3 The CT scan demonstrates a mass in the head of the pancreas. The scan is performed to assess local invasion. In this case there is no obvious disruption of tissue planes or evidence of portal vein invasion and no obvious lymph node metastases. A metallic stent is seen within the CBD.

43.4 Important aetiological factors for the development of pancreatic cancer are: smoking (relative risk 2); high dietary fat intake (Japan, relative risk 4); diabetes mellitus (relative risk 2); familial adenomatous polyposis.

43.5 A laparotomy should be performed and the pancreas and surrounding anatomy explored. If the tumour is small with no local invasion or lymphadenopathy a Whipple's procedure should be performed. This is *en bloc* removal of the gallbladder, common bile duct, duodenum, head of pancreas with or without the pylorus. If there is evidence of portal vein invasion or metastases then a biliary-enteric bypass (cholecystojejunostomy or choledochojejunostomy) and gastroenterostomy should be performed. For patients with curative resections the survival at 5 years is 20–25%. For other patients the mean survival is 6–9 months.

Case 44 – Gallbladder carcinoma

44.1 There is a polypoid lesion arising from the wall of the gallbladder. Unlike gallstones it does not cast an acoustic shadow.

44.2 Following a staging CT, the patient should undergo a laparotomy with a view to cholecystectomy. Gallbladder carcinomas spread via blood and lymphatics and also directly into the liver and at the time of presentation the tumour is often too advanced for curative surgery. In such a situation a choledochojejunostomy should be performed to bypass the obstruction. If surgery is not possible the biliary tree should be stented to alleviate symptoms.

44.3 The prognosis is poor, with more than 90% of patients dying within 1 year of diagnosis.

44.4 The ERCP demonstrates a high obstruction of the common bile duct. In Figure 44c a drain has been placed across the obstructing lesion to allow relief of jaundice.

44.5 If a tumour is identified at the time of a laparoscopic cholecystectomy, the procedure should be converted to an open procedure since there have been several reports of abdominal wall recurrence when tumours have been removed laparoscopically. The need for further treatment will depend on tumour stage. If the lesion is a T1 tumour then no further treatment is required. Tumours of T2 status should be referred to a hepatobiliary surgeon for further resection of the extra-hepatic biliary tree together with segments 4 and 5 of the liver with hepaticojejunostomy reconstruction.

Lower gastrointestinal

Case 45 – Crohn's disease

45.1 Figure 45a is a double-contrast (air and barium) barium enema showing irregularity of the mucosa of the terminal ileum. Figure 45b shows a segment of strictured rectum with evidence of fistula formation. Figure 45c shows a probe passing through a fistula-in-ano. These are characteristic features of Crohn's disease.

45.2 Crohn's disease is a disease of Caucasians, notably in Northern Europe (UK and Scandinavia) and North America. It has a higher incidence in Jewish populations, and a lower incidence in Asia, Africa and Southern Europe. The disease has a bimodal age distribution, one in the 20–40 age-group and one in the 60–70 age-group. 10% of patients have a first-degree family member affected. Smokers have a higher incidence than non-smokers, and partners of index cases have a slightly higher risk compared with the general population. Males and females are affected equally. Crohn's disease and ulcerative colitis have many epidemiological features in common.

45.3 Figure 45d shows the microscopy of a mesenteric lymph node with evidence of epithelioid granuloma formation, the histopathologic hallmark of Crohn's disease. Granulomas are found in approximately 60% of patients. They may be found at any layer in the bowel wall and in the regional lymph nodes. They become less common as the duration of disease increases and are more numerous in the distal bowel, i.e. they are most common in the rectum.

45.4 The two main complications of Crohn's disease are obstruction and fistulation. Others include bleeding, perforation, malignant change and malabsorption.

45.5 Approximately 70% of patients will ultimately undergo surgery. The two main operations employed are resection and strictureplasty.

Case 46 – Ulcerative colitis

46.1 Ulcerative colitis presenting as toxic megacolon.

46.2 No. Only 5% of patients with ulcerative colitis present in this way. Toxic megacolon can occur in Crohn's disease (less common than in ulcerative colitis), and infective colitis.

46.3 The extra-intestinal manifestations can be divided into those related to the intestinal disease activity: pyoderma gangrenosum, erythema nodosum, aphthous ulcers of the mouth and vagina, iritis and large joint arthritis. Those unrelated to the intestinal disease activity are: sacroiliitis, ankylosing spondylitis, chronic active hepatitis, cirrhosis, sclerosing cholangitis, cholangiocarcinoma, fingernail clubbing.

46.4 The main complications are perforation, bleeding and malignant change (risk greater than in Crohn's disease). The risk of malignancy increases as the extent and duration of disease increase.

46.5 The treatment of toxic megacolon is panproctocolectomy. In an elective setting acute exacerbations of ulcerative colitis are managed medically with corticosteroids and azathioprine. If the disease is limited to the rectum steroid enemas may be used. Once remission is achieved salicylic acid derivatives are used for maintenance therapy. The surgical treatment of ulcerative colitis is colectomy. The operations can be divided into three types:

1 panproctocolectomy with ileostomy – disadvantage is that a young patient is left with a stoma;

2 subtotal colectomy and ileorectal anastomosis – this is appropriate if the rectum is only mildly affected. The disadvantage is that there is a high relapse rate due to persisting disease in the rectum, often requiring conversion to ileostomy;

3 restorative proctocolectomy – a subtotal colectomy is performed and the rectum transected at the level of the pelvic floor. The remaining rectal mucosa is stripped from the underlying tissue, and a reservoir pouch constructed from ileum anastomosed onto the denuded rectum. Various pouch configurations exist. They are named after the letter they resemble (S, J, H, W).

Case 47 – Acute appendicitis

47.1 Acute appendicitis. This is the classical description of appendicitis, occurring in approximately half of patients. Initially the pain is poorly localised to the periumbilical region as a result of irritation of the visceral peritoneum. Later as the parietal peritoneum becomes involved in the inflammatory process the pain is more localised.

47.2 The following groups of patients have a higher morbidity and mortality: the young (<5 years), the elderly, pregnant females, neutropenic patients. In infants less than 1 year of age the incidence of perforation is close to 100%, in those under 2 it is 70–80%. It remains more than 50% up to age 5. The higher morbidity and mortality in this group is due to the delay in diagnosis and the incomplete development of the omentum, preventing the containment of peritonitis. In the elderly appendicitis not uncommonly presents as small bowel obstruction due to inflammatory adhesive bands. In pregnancy the incidence of premature labour is approximately 50% in the third trimester for those developing appendicitis.

47.3 Appendicectomy is being carried out laparoscopically. The patient is most likely to be a female of child-bearing age. The clinical diagnosis of acute appendicitis is incorrect in 15–20% of patients, evidenced by normal appendiceal histology. The chances of this occurring are greater in young females (30–45%) as gynaecologic causes of right iliac fossa pain are common in this group. In this group diagnostic laparoscopy may be used. If acute appendicitis is confirmed depending upon the surgeon's preference appendicectomy can be performed laparoscopically or the procedure converted to an open appendicectomy.

47.4 Charles McBurney (1845–1913) and Thorkild Rovsing (1862–1937). McBurney's point is a point 1.5–2.0 inches along a line joining the anterior superior iliac spine and the umbilicus. It is the point of maximal tenderness in acute appendicitis. Rovsing's sign is the elicitation of right iliac fossa pain on palpating the left iliac fossa. This is presumed to be due to a shift to the right of loops of small bowel that then impinge upon the inflamed appendix.

47.5 Carcinoid tumour and adenocarcinoma.

Case 48 – Meckel's diverticulum

48.1 Meckel's diverticulum. This is a remnant of the vitello-intestinal (omphalomesenteric) duct, normally obliterated in the 7th week *in utero*.

48.2 Technetium scan. ^{99m}Tc-pertechnetate is taken up by gastric mucosa, and thus only in those patients in whom the Meckel's diverticulum contains actively bleeding ectopic gastric mucosa will it prove useful.

48.3 It is present in 2% of the population, and is symptomatic in 30% of these.

48.4 The most common complications in order of frequency are bleeding, intestinal obstruction (due to volvulus, intussusception, or incarceration of the diverticulum in a hernia), diverticulitis and perforation.

48.5 If a Meckel's diverticulum is discovered incidentally during the course of a laparotomy for another pathology it should be left alone. For symptomatic patients the treatment is either diverticulectomy or segmental resection, the choice depending upon the size of the diverticulum, and the presence or absence of ectopic gastric mucosa. In the presence of ectopic gastric or pancreatic mucosa resection is the best option.

Case 49 – Diverticular disease

49.1 Figure 49a shows a double-contrast barium enema with diverticular disease of the sigmoid colon. Figure 49b shows a sigmoid colectomy specimen affected by diverticular disease.

49.2 The pathological features of diverticular disease are a thickening of the circular and longitudinal layers of the muscularis propria. Diverticular disease may affect any site in the colon except the appendix and rectum, which lack taeniae coli. The most commonly affected site is the sigmoid colon, which is involved as the sole site in more than 75% of cases and is affected overall in more than 90% of all cases.

49.3 The investigations shown are a double-contrast barium enema (Figure 49c) and contrast-enhanced computerised tomography (Figure 49d). The complication shown is a para-colic abscess with fistula. Other complications of diverticular disease are diverticulitis, bleeding, peritonitis and intestinal obstruction.

49.4 The diverticula are not true diverticula. They are false diverticula, i.e. protrusions of mucosa and submucosa through the muscularis propria. True diverticula are congenital in origin and are lined by all layers of the bowel wall.

49.5 The incidence of diverticular disease is closely related to age, being <5% at age 40, 30% by age 60 and up to 65% by age 85 years. Males and females are affected equally. It is common in North America, Western Europe and Australia/New Zealand, and uncommon in Africa, South America and Asia.

Case 50 – Small bowel obstruction

50.1 Plain abdominal radiographs, erect (Figure 50a) and supine (Figure 50b) films, showing dilated small bowel loops and multiple air-fluid levels. The findings indicate small bowel obstruction.

50.2 The per-operative photograph shows strangulation of the small bowel. The congested appearance is due to venous ischaemia. In this case a small bowel volvulus occurred around an omental band.

50.3 In the UK the most common three causes of small bowel obstruction in adults are adhesions, incarcerated hernias and small bowel tumours.

50.4 The management depends upon whether or not the patient has signs of perforation or peritonitis. In the absence of these the management is conservative, i.e. intravenous fluid and electrolyte replacement, insertion of nasogastric and urinary catheter, and careful observation. If the situation does not settle within 48 hours or the patient develops signs of peritonitis, laparotomy should be performed. Approximately 50% of patients with adhesive small bowel obstruction settle on conservative therapy. The need for surgical intervention is more likely in a patient who has not undergone any prior abdominal surgery.

50.5 A barium meal and follow-through.

Case 51 – Adenocarcinoma of the colon

51.1 Gastroscopy to look for upper gastrointestinal causes of anaemia, and either barium enema or colonoscopy to look for lower gastrointestinal causes of anaemia.

51.2 Double-contrast barium enema (Figure 51a). It shows a filling defect in the transverse colon (the classic apple-core lesion) consistent with adenocarcinoma of the colon.

51.3 The tumour is close to the hepatic flexure and can thus be managed by either an extended right hemicolectomy (resection of 10–15 cm of terminal ileum, the caecum, the ascending colon and the transverse colon) or a transverse colectomy (resection of transverse colon alone).

51.4 Dukes' classification of rectal carcinoma, now applied to all colorectal carcinomas, is a pathologic staging of the disease. It may be used as a prognostic indicator for the disease. A Dukes' A carcinoma is one confined to the bowel with no evidence of metastatic tumour in the regional lymph nodes. Dukes' B carcinoma is a tumour that extends through the full thickness of the bowel wall with no evidence of metastatic tumour in the regional lymph nodes. Dukes' C carcinoma is one associated with metastatic tumour in the regional lymph nodes, irrespective of the bowel wall tumour depth. The 5 year survival for the three stages is 95%, 70% and 35% respectively. In the UK the proportion of tumours by Dukes' stage is 15%, 35% and 50%. Although not described in the original classification, a Dukes' D stage is taken to be synonymous with distant (haematogenous) metastases.

51.5 Cutaneous metastases in a laparotomy scar.

Case 52 – Haemorrhoids

52.1 Thrombosed haemorrhoids.

52.2 Bleeding.

52.3 Treatment of thrombosed haemorrhoids is either conservative (ice-packs and analgesia) or haemorrhoidectomy. Most cases resolve with conservative therapy. The disadvantage of emergency surgery is distortion of the anatomy by oedema and the higher risk of iatrogenic damage to the anal sphincter. The elective treatment of haemorrhoids is tailored according to the severity of the condition. First degree haemorrhoids (bleed but do not prolapse) are managed by prescribing fybogel or adhering to a high fibre diet. Second degree haemorrhoids (prolapse with defaecation but then reduce spontaneously) are managed by either injection sclerotherapy (5% phenol in arachis oil) or elastic band ligation. Third degree haemorrhoids (prolapse and require manual reduction) are managed by haemorrhoidectomy. With sclerotherapy, sclerosant is injected into the submucosa so that a bleb is raised. 1–2 mL are sufficient per haemorrhoid. No more than three should be treated at a single visit. The most popular haemorrhoidectomy technique in the UK is the Milligan–Morgan haemorrhoidectomy which is a ligation and excision technique.

52.4 It is important to inject the haemorrhoids or band them well above the squamous epithelium. The mucosa below the squamo-columnar junction is sensitive to touch and thus injection or banding at this level will be painful.

52.5 Post-operatively a faecal softener is prescribed as defaecation is painful until the area has healed.

Case 53 – Adenocarcinoma of the rectum

53.1 The plain abdominal radiograph (Figure 53a) shows distended loops of large bowel with absence of gas below the descending colon consistent with an obstructing lesion in the rectosigmoid. The resection specimen (Figure 53b) shows an adenocarcinoma of the rectum.

53.2 This gentleman can be managed in one of several ways:

1 Hartmann's procedure;

2 on-table lavage, resection and primary anastomosis, possibly with covering stoma;

3 total colectomy – if the caecum is markedly distended and shows signs of impending perforation this is the best option.

For the elective treatment a small proportion of early rectal cancers (Dukes' A) can be treated by transanal resection. In general however the two operations employed are anterior resection and abdominoperineal resection. In the latter the proximal sigmoid colon is brought out as a permanent colostomy. In the former bowel continuity is restored by end-to-end anastomosis.

The choice of procedure depends upon the distal extent of the tumour. In general, abdominoperineal excision of the rectum is required for lesions 5 cm or less from the anal verge. Approximately 75% of rectal cancers can be treated by anterior resection.

53.3 The investigations shown are an ultrasound scan of the liver (Figure 53c) showing a solitary liver metastasis and a contrast-enhanced CT scan of the abdomen (Figure 53d) showing a solitary liver metastasis and thickening of the omentum as a result of tumour infiltration.

53.4 The indications for hepatic resection are physiological fitness for surgery, less than four metastases confined to one hepatic lobe and no evidence of locally recurrent disease.

53.5 5-Fluorouracil. It is given intravenously as its absorption from the gut is unreliable due to a high hepatic first-pass effect. Adverse effects include oral ulceration, diarrhoea and myelo-suppression. Rarer adverse effects include megaloblastic anaemia and cerebellar ataxia.

Case 54 – Familial adenomatous polyposis

54.1 Familial adenomatous polyposis.

54.2 Autosomal dominant, with the gene located on the short arm of chromosome 5. The incidence is approximately 1 in 10 000 liveborn.

54.3 Associated features include hamartomas of the stomach, duodenal adenomas, osteomas of the mandible, dental cysts, epidermoid cysts, retinal pigmentation and desmoid tumours.

54.4 Treatment involves prophylactic removal of the entire colon. This is achieved by either subtotal colectomy and ileorectal anastomosis or restorative proctocolectomy. The former has the disadvantage of requiring regular sigmoidoscopic follow-up with the risk that future completion proctectomy will be necessary.

54.5 Duodenal adenocarcinoma. Surveillance gastroscopy is required to detect duodenal adenomas before malignant change occurs.

Case 55 – Colonic volvulus

55.1 Erect (Figure 55a) and supine (Figure 55b) plain abdominal radiographs showing a caecal volvulus. Air-fluid levels are evident in Figure 55a.

55.2 The organ must have a mesentery. A volvulus is a rotation of an organ around its mesentery.

55.3 No. Volvulus most commonly affects the sigmoid colon (75% of cases). Other segments of the colon that may be affected are the transverse colon and the splenic flexure. Extra-colonic volvulus may affect the stomach, gallbladder and small bowel.

55.4 It is an uncommon cause of large bowel obstruction in the Western World. It is common however in Africa and parts of Eastern Europe and Asia. In the Western World the disease is associated with chronic constipation. Many patients have associated neurological or psychiatric diseases, which as a consequence of the disease itself or its treatment result in poor bowel motility. Outside the Western World it is thought to result from a redundant sigmoid colon due to a high-fibre diet. In the West the patients tend to be elderly and of both sexes, while in the Eastern World and Africa they are middle-aged males.

55.5 The management of the patient depends upon whether or not there are signs of perforation or peritonitis. In the absence of these features the condition can be managed conservatively by sigmoidoscopy and placement of a rectal tube to deflate the distended bowel. The patient later undergoes elective resection. If there are signs of perforation or peritonitis emergency laparotomy should be undertaken. Treatment should be operative detorsion and either resection or fixation of the affected segment of colon.

Case 56 – Anorectal sepsis

56.1 Perianal abscess in a child (Figure 56a) and ischiorectal abscess in an adult (Figure 56b).

56.2 Features that suggest the presence of a fistula-in-ano are a history of recurrent episodes of anorectal sepsis and the isolation of gastrointestinal pathogens (rather than skin pathogens) from the abscess fluid.

56.3 The disease is more common in males with a peak incidence between the ages of 20–40 years. Up to 5% of patients have associated disease, most commonly Crohn's disease or diabetes mellitus.

56.4 The management of anorectal sepsis is abscess incision and drainage combined with examination under anaesthetic and sigmoidoscopy. Fistulas are found in association with perianal abscesses in up to 25% of patients. If the fistula is intersphincteric the management includes fistulotomy; this is accomplished either as part of a one-stage procedure or a delayed procedure after 7–10 days. Suprasphincteric fistulas are managed by seton insertion. A seton is a length of knotted monofilament nylon passed through the fistula tract. It should not be tied too tightly and remains in place for several months. Its mode of action is to gradually 'cheese-wire' through the tissues, permitting healing proximal to and cutting distal to its location.

56.5 Goodsall's rule describes the usual relationship of internal and external fistula orifices. To understand it assume that the patient is lying supine with an imaginary horizontal line drawn through the midpoint of the anal canal. An external opening anterior to this line will have an internal opening that follows a straight radial tract. An external opening posterior to this line will have a tract that pursues a horseshoe-shaped tract and an internal opening in the midline posteriorly.

Case 57 – Vesicocolic fistula

57.1 A double-contrast barium enema showing passage of barium from the sigmoid colon into the bladder. The patient has a vesicocolic fistula.

57.2 The classical presenting features are pneumaturia and faecaluria (up to 80%). Other features include bladder-irritative symptoms in 50% (frequency, urgency, dysuria) and fever/chills (35%). The passage of urine per rectum is rare (8%) because of the higher colonic pressure relative to the intravesical pressure. It may occur following colostomy formation and in patients with severe bladder outflow obstruction. A palpable abdominal mass is present in one-third of patients. Urinalysis may show the findings of a urinary tract infection, particulate matter or rhabdomyocytes derived from undigested meat residue in the stool.

57.3 The causes of vesicocolic fistula can be divided into four categories:

1 inflammatory – diverticulitis, inflammatory bowel disease, pelvic sepsis from other causes, tuberculosis, actinomycosis;

2 neoplastic – adenocarcinomas of the rectosigmoid and cervix;

3 traumatic – pelvic fractures, penetrating injuries, following transurethral or open prostatectomy;

4 following radiotherapy to the pelvis.

Diverticulitis (50%), inflammatory bowel disease (20%) and malignancy (20%) account for most cases.

57.4 Colovesical fistula secondary to diverticulitis occurs up to five times more commonly in males than females. The intervening uterus in females is thought to lessen the chances of fistulation to the bladder. Females develop colovaginal fistulas seven times more commonly than colovesical fistulas. Of the females developing colovesical fistulas secondary to diverticulitis a high proportion have undergone prior hysterectomy.

57.5 The treatment depends upon the underlying cause and the general health of the patient. In debilitated patients with advanced malignancy a defunctioning colostomy may be the best option. Most patients will however require surgical repair. This is achieved by *en bloc* resection of the affected segment of bowel and bladder. Bowel continuity is restored by primary anastomosis and the bladder repaired. When possible, omentum should be sutured over the surface of the bladder to prevent subsequent apposition of the colon and bladder.

Case 58 – Mesenteric vascular occlusion

58.1 The diagnosis is small bowel gangrene as a result of acute mesenteric arterial occlusion.

58.2 The causes of small bowel arterial infarction are:

1 superior mesenteric artery occlusion – atheromatous occlusion (usually affecting the main trunk of the artery);

2 superior mesenteric artery emboli (95% in association with atrial fibrillation). Emboli usually impact just beyond the middle colic branch of the SMA resulting in a sparing of the upper jejunum and transverse colon;

3 low-output states – cardiac failure, hypovolaemic shock (blood loss, septicaemia), splanchnic vasoconstriction, drugs (vasopressin, adrenaline, noradrenaline), trauma.

58.3 All forms of acute occlusion produce similar signs. Clinical features are severe abdominal pain often disproportionate to the scanty physical signs, a profound leucocytosis (often >20 000 leucocytes per mm^3), vomiting, diarrhoea, pyrexia, oliguria and acidosis. Later melaena develops in association with peritonitis, and ultimately death from septicaemia.

58.4 The mucosa is the most sensitive to ischaemia. Infarction occurs from the mucosa outwards.

58.5 When the mainstem of the SMA is occluded a catastrophic infarction of the intestine occurs from a point just beyond the duodenojejunal flexure to the splenic flexure of the colon. The management options are:

1 embolectomy, revascularisation and resection of ischaemic bowel;

2 palliation (no resection) in the elderly. Extensive resection is likely to leave the patient dependent upon total parenteral nutrition.

Case 59 – Rectal prolapse

59.1 Complete rectal prolapse. The patient has been managed by a DeLorme's procedure.

59.2 Complete rectal prolapse (all layers of the gut) is a condition affecting principally elderly females (M:F 1:20). Partial rectal prolapse (mucosa only) occurs throughout the first year of life and affects male and female infants equally.

59.3 Predisposing factors in children include poor toilet training, constipation or diarrhoea. Paroxysms of coughing can result in a partial rectal prolapse. In adults the cause is believed to be a weakness of the anal sphincter and pelvic floor. Anorectal manometry on patients with rectal prolapse reveals a reduction in resting anal pressure and maximum voluntary contraction pressure.

59.4 50% of adult patients have some degree of faecal incontinence.

59.5 Infants are managed by correct bowel training. The child should be toileted at regular intervals to prevent excessive straining with prescription of a mild laxative if necessary. Refractory cases can be managed by submucosal injection of sclerosant. In adults minor mucosal prolapse can be managed by submucosal injection of sclerosant. Surgical repair is necessary for complete rectal prolapse. There are many different ways of achieving this. In general they are divided into perineal (DeLorme's procedure, perineal rectosigmoidectomy) and abdominal rectopexy procedures.

Case 60 – Fissure-in-ano

60.1 Fissure-in-ano.

60.2 The condition is more common in males than females. Peak incidence is between the ages of 20–30 years. 90% of fissures are located at the posterior anal margin. Anterior fissures are more common in females and may follow childbirth (vaginal delivery).

60.3 The management of an acute anal fissure is conservative – topical lignocaine gel for its analgesic effect and the prescription of a faecal softener. After resolution a high fibre diet may reduce the risk of recurrence. The principal of management of a chronic anal fissure is to reduce internal anal sphincter spasm. This is achieved by either anal dilatation or internal sphincterotomy (lateral or posterior). Recent work has indicated that topical nitrates (GTN) will heal chronic anal fissures. The aetiology of chronic anal fissure is believed to be ischaemia secondary to sphincter spasm. Nitrates exert a local vasodilator effect and thus permit healing.

60.4 The main complications are treatment failure and faecal incontinence.

60.5 Lateral sphincterotomy is the treatment of choice. It may be performed by either a closed or an open technique. Anal dilatation results in an uncontrolled disruption of the internal anal sphincter and thus its reproducibility from one occasion to the next is poor. High rates of faecal incontinence have been reported. Lateral sphincterotomy results in a controlled surgical division of the sphincter. Posterior sphincterotomy has a higher rate of faecal incontinence than lateral sphincterotomy.

Case 61 – Enteral nutrition

61.1 Feeding jejunostomy.

61.2 Patients undergoing major upper gastrointestinal surgery, patients undergoing laparotomy after major trauma and patients who may receive radiochemotherapy following surgery.

61.3 Percutaneous endoscopic gastrostomy.

61.4 This is particularly useful for long-term feeding in patients with neurological disabilities (especially stroke patients) who have swallowing difficulties. In it also useful in patients with head and neck malignancies undergoing surgery and in children with growth problems or high calorie requirements (cystic fibrosis).

61.5 The main complications are:

1 tube-related (malposition, blockage);

2 diet-related (diarrhoea, bloating, nausea, colicky abdominal pain);

3 metabolic/biochemical (hypoglycaemia, hyperglycaemia, electrolyte disorder, vitamin and mineral deficiency);

4 cellulitis of the skin around the tube.

Case 62 – Radiation injury to the small bowel

62.1 Radiotherapy. Figure 62 shows a segment of small intestine with two areas of stricturing as a late consequence of irradiation injury. Any factors that increase the risk of adhesions predispose to intestinal injury – prior operations, sepsis. Certain chemotherapeutic agents (doxorubicin, 5-fluourouracil and actinomycin D) act as radiation sensitisers and exacerbate the effects of therapeutic radiotherapy.

62.2 Radiotherapy is given as a primary treatment to certain patients with adenocarcinomas of the endometrium and prostate and transitional cell carcinoma of the bladder. It may be given as adjuvant therapy to patients with adenocarcinomas of the large bowel, ovary, cervix, germ cell tumours of the testis and lymphomas.

62.3 Such stricturing is due to the effects of irradiation on nutrient blood vessels. There is a progressive obliterative vasculitis resulting in tissue hypoxia and fibrosis. Some patients are asymptomatic for long periods of time before developing symptoms of chronic intestinal injury; others progress from a symptomatic acute injury state to a symptomatic chronic state.

62.4 At therapeutic doses many patients experience no gastrointestinal upset at all. Others may experience transient symptoms such as diarrhoea, steatorrhoea, crampy abdominal pain and nausea/vomiting. Treatment is supportive whilst the adverse effects last.

62.5 Diagnosis is based upon a history suggestive of chronic or recurrent small bowel obstruction in a patient previously treated with radiotherapy. Appropriate imaging would be a barium meal and follow-through. In general the treatment is surgical resection of the affected segment of small bowel with an anastomosis between two segments of normal-appearing intestine. Acute exacerbations in some patients may respond to conservative measures such as nasogastric suction, intravenous fluids and corticosteroids.

Case 63 – Squamous cell carcinoma of the anus

63.1 Squamous cell (epidermoid) carcinoma of the anus.

63.2 It is customary to divide anal carcinoma into two main types based upon the site of origin, that arising from the anal canal and that arising from the anal margin. This distinction is important in relation to both treatment and prognosis. Carcinoma arising from the anal margin accounts for around 25% of tumours. It is more commonly seen in females. Anal canal carcinoma accounts for 75% of tumours and is more commonly seen in males (M:F 4:1). The more proximal the tumour the more poorly differentiated it is and the lower the chance that it will show keratinisation. Thus, most anal margin tumours produce keratin but only one-third of canal tumours do. Tumours of the upper anal canal are usually basaloid or cloacogenic, that is they demonstrate evidence of origin from the transitional zone of epithelium.

63.3 Risk factors for the development of anal carcinoma are infection with human papilloma virus, in particular type 16 (common in homosexuals), leukoplakia, perianal Crohn's disease and fistula-in-ano.

63.4 The usual presenting features are pain and bleeding. Uncommonly metastatic superficial inguinal lymphadenopathy is the first presentation.

63.5 The treatment of anal margin cancers is local excision. For anal canal tumours appropriate therapy is either abdominoperineal excision of the rectum or radiotherapy. When radiotherapy is used it is usually given in conjunction with adjuvant chemotherapy (mitomycin C and 5-fluorouracil). The general trend is towards employing radiochemotherapy as the primary treatment so that preservation of sphincter function can be achieved.

Breast

Case 64 – Breast abscess

64.1 There is a tense erythematous swelling of the right breast.

64.2 The likely diagnosis is a breast abscess. An important differential, especially in older ladies, is inflammatory breast carcinoma which has an identical mode of presentation.

64.3 The group classically said to develop breast abscesses are lactating mothers (80% of all breast abscesses). It is believed that infection develops in cracks in the nipple. Abscesses are most commonly seen in the first month post-partum.

64.4 The most common organism isolated is *Staphylococcus aureus*. Others include streptococci, enterococci and anaerobes.

64.5 An incision large enough to ensure adequate abscess cavity drainage is made and all loculi interrupted. It is important to send a sample of pus to microbiology and any suspicious tissue for histological examination. Following irrigation, the cavity is packed with a suitable material such as Kaltostat and left to heal by secondary intention.

Case 65 – Fibroadenoma

65.1 This is a breast ultrasound and demonstrates a well-defined, hypo-echoic mass with post-acoustic enhancement. These appearances are characteristic of a fibroadenoma.

65.2 Fibroadenomas are well-circumscribed, firm, smooth, mobile and almond-shaped.

65.3 Fibroadenomas are the most common breast lumps in women <35 years but may occur at any age from menarche to menopause. Giant fibroadenomas (>5 cm) occur in a younger age group and are common in Africa.

65.4 Fibroadenomas are now regarded as being aberrations of normal breast tissue development and not true tumours. However, there appears to be a small risk of carcinomatous transformation of 1 per 1000.

65.5 Treatment of fibroadenomas may be non-operative or operative. If the diagnosis is confirmed by ultrasound and FNA the patient can be reassured. Anxious patients may opt for a lumpectomy.

Case 66 – Cystic breast disease

66.1 There are multiple opacities in both breasts each of which is surrounded by a halo. This is the characteristic appearance of cystic breast disease.

66.2 The majority of women present with a breast lump and one-third will report pain. Cystic disease is a common condition and approximately 7% of all women present with this condition. The cysts are single in 50%, one-third have 2–5 cysts and the remainder develop >5 cysts. One-third have bilateral disease.

66.3 Cystic disease is believed to represent an involutional process within the breast, hence its perimenopausal presentation.

66.4 This patient is having a cyst aspirated. If the aspirate is blood-stained it should be sent for cytological examination. The breast should be re-examined post-aspiration to exclude an associated carcinoma.

66.5 Patients should be re-examined after 1 month. If the cyst has recurred a further aspiration should be performed. Cysts that re-accumulate rapidly after a second aspiration should be excised as there may be an associated carcinoma. Patients with recurrent cystic disease may also benefit from treatment with danazol.

Case 67 – Paget's disease

67.1 There is an erythematous, eczematous lesion affecting the nipple and areola of the left breast.

67.2 Paget's disease of the nipple. (n.b. Paget's is usually unilateral whereas eczema is bilateral).

67.3 Paget's disease is due to invasion of the nipple by malignant cells from an underlying neoplasm. Examination will reveal a palpable mass in 50% of cases. 60% will have palpable nodal disease. Of those with no obvious mass, careful cytological study of biopsies will invariably reveal a ductal carcinoma *in situ* (DCIS) or invasive ductal carcinoma.

67.4 Paget's disease may be seen in the genital region, perineum and axillae. Extramammary Paget's is less commonly associated with an underlying neoplasm than mammary Paget's.

67.5 If an invasive tumour is identified the patient should be offered mastectomy with axillary dissection. Patients with no obvious mass will probably have DCIS and should be offered either mastectomy or alternatively cone excision of the nipple/areola complex followed by radiotherapy.

Case 68 – Nipple discharge

68.1 The differential diagnosis of a bloody discharge includes duct papilloma, duct ectasia, fibroadenosis or carcinoma. An underlying malignancy is identified in 20–30% of cases.

68.2 If a single papilloma is identified a microdochectomy should be performed. However, when the duct of origin is uncertain, all major ducts should be excised (Hadfield's operation).

68.3 Duct ectasia.

68.4 Duct ectasia is a benign condition in which the subareolar ducts are dilated and become filled with inspissated material. Chronic inflammation may lead to nipple retraction.

68.5 Surgery is indicated only if there is associated nipple retraction or troublesome discharge. The radiological features of ectasia may mimic a carcinoma with retroareolar thickening of the ducts together with microcalcification. An excision biopsy may be necessary for this reason. Operative options are the same as for a papilloma.

Case 69 – Gynaecomastia

69.1 Bilateral gynaecomastia.

69.2 The common underlying cause for all cases of gynaecomastia is an imbalance between oestrogen and androgen levels.

69.3 I Physiological – small peak in infants which usually resolves by 6 months of age; large peak around puberty which affects up to 70% of males – usually resolves within 2 years when adult testosterone levels are reached; senile peak which affects 35% of the adult male population and is related to reduced testosterone levels.

II Secondary – reduced testosterone (castration, orchitis, hypogonadism, Klinefelter's syndrome); increased oestrogen (testicular and adrenal tumours, hepatoma, ectopic hormone production) and drug-induced (oestrogens, cyproterone, cimetidine, digoxin, cannabis, phenothiazines, tricyclic antidepressants, methyldopa, metoclopramide, isoniazid, opiates, anabolic steroids).

69.4 Patients, in particular the elderly with long-standing gynaecomastia, should undergo mammography with FNA of any suspicious lesions.

69.5 Patients with physiological gynaecomastia should be reassured that their condition will resolve. Patients with secondary gynaecomastia usually resolve with cessation of relevant drug therapy. If breast tenderness is the most troublesome factor the anti-gonadotrophin danazol may be effective whilst subcutaneous mastectomy may be performed for cosmetic reasons in adult patients. Adult patients should be examined to exclude associated breast cancer.

Case 70 – Ductal carcinoma *in situ*

70.1 This is a cranial-caudal mammogram demonstrating widespread microcalcification in keeping with ductal carcinoma *in situ*.

70.2 Prior to the advent of breast screening the incidence of DCIS in symptomatic patients was believed to be 5%. In the screened population it now represents 20–30% of detected lesions.

70.3 Figure 70b is a radiograph of a wide local excision specimen and demonstrates an area of microcalcification in the centre of the specimen. It is important to orientate the specimen following excision so as to allow the pathologist to comment on completeness of excision.

70.4 The need for further treatment is controversial and is the subject of a large multicentre trial (DCIS trial) which is assessing the role of adjuvant radiotherapy and tamoxifen following complete excision of the DCIS. If the initial excision is incomplete, a further excision should be performed. For patients with multifocal disease, a mastectomy may be appropriate.

70.5 Approximately 25% of patients have an incomplete primary excision and require further local excision. If left untreated approximately one-third develop an ipsilateral breast cancer. However, the incidence of metastases is low and the incidence of nodal involvement is less than 1%.

Case 71 – Screen-detected breast cancer

71.1 Figure 71a is a cranial-caudal view and 71b is an oblique view. They demonstrate a small lesion in the upper outer quadrant of the right breast.

71.2 This ultrasound shows that the mass is solid with an irregular outline. This is the typical appearance of a carcinoma.

71.3 Since the mass is not palpable a hand-guided fine needle aspiration is not possible. In this case an ultrasound-guided biopsy could be performed. An alternative for small, deep lesions would be an X-ray-guided stereotactic biopsy.

71.4 C1 = inadequate specimen
C2 = benign cells
C3 = atypia, probably benign
C4 = suspicious of malignancy
C5 = malignant cells

71.5 This patient has undergone a wire-localisation biopsy. This technique is used for small non-palpable lesions. A hooked-wire is inserted under ultrasound or X-ray control by a radiologist. The patient is then taken to theatre and the tissue around the tip of the wire is excised and sent for pathological examination. A repeat X-ray is taken of the specimen to ensure that the suspicious area has been completely excised.

Case 72 – Breast cancer

72.1 It shows an irregular non-homogenous mass with a spiculated border. Areas of microcalcification are also noted within the mass. These features are typical of carcinoma.

72.2 A woman's lifetime risk for developing breast cancer is 1 in 12 and the disease carries an annual mortality in the UK of 13 000. The incidence in males is 1/100th that of females.

72.3 The factors which are associated with an increased risk of breast cancer are: previous breast carcinoma, family history of breast carcinoma, female gender, and age >50 years. Other factors include a history of benign breast disease, advanced age at first pregnancy, early menarche, use of contraceptive pill, late menopause, use of hormone replacement therapy, and ionising radiation.

72.4 Breast cancer is classified according to the TNM classification in which T represents the size of the primary tumour, N corresponds to regional lymph nodes and M to the presence or absence of distant metastases.

    T1   <2 cm

    T2   2–5 cm

    T3   >5 cm

T4a Involvement of chest wall

T4b Involvement of skin (ulceration, infiltration, peau d'orange and satellite nodules)

T4c a and b together

T4d Inflammatory cancer

N0 No regional node metastasis

N1 Mobile ipsilateral nodes

N2 Fixed ipsilateral nodes

N3 Internal mammary node involvement

M0 No diastant metastasis

M1 Distant metastasis (including ipsilateral supraclavicular)

72.5 Patients with small tumours and no evidence of lymph node or distant metastases may be treated equally successfully by mastectomy or wide local excision with axillary clearance. Long-term disease free survival for such a patient is in the order of 80–90% whereas a patient with a similar-sized tumour but positive nodes would have a predicted 5-year survival of <50%.

Case 73 – Locally advanced breast cancer

73.1 There is marked distortion and destruction of the left breast with puckering of the skin and erosion of the nipple by a malignant ulcer.

73.2 Fungating breast carcinoma.

73.3 The contralateral breast, both axillae and cervical regions should be examined for assessment of local disease. Examination of the abdomen (hepatomegaly or ascites), chest (metastases or pleural effusion) and axial skeleton (bony tenderness) to exclude distant metastases.

73.4 The aim of treatment is to obtain local control of the disease. The simplest treatment is 20 mg per day of tamoxifen which has an overall response rate of around 30%. Surgery in the form of toilet mastectomy removes the tumour completely but is a major operation. Some benefit has been shown from the use of chemo-radiotherapy consisting of three courses of doxorubicin and vincristine at 3 week intervals followed by radical radiotherapy.

73.5 The overall 5-year survival rate for such a lesion is around 5%.

Case 74 – Metastatic breast carcinoma

74.1 There is local recurrence of the breast cancer.

74.2 The diagnosis may be confirmed by obtaining either FNA or Tru-cut biopsy.

74.3 The radiograph demonstrates multiple metastases distributed throughout both lung fields.

74.4 The important problems of metastatic disease include adequate pain control, persistent hypercalcaemia, pathological fractures, cerebral metastases and superior vena caval obstruction.

74.5 The primary treatment of breast carcinoma, metastatic to the lungs is systemic chemotherapy. Other measures include:

1 pain control with opioids and NSAIDS;
2 correction of hypercalcaemia with hydration, corticosteroids or biphosphonates;
3 radiotherapy to painful skeletal metastases;
4 internal fixation of long bones for pathological fractures;
5 corticosteroids for cerebral metastases;
6 radiotherapy for superior vena caval obstruction secondary to malignant lymphadenopathy.

Case 75 – Cystosarcoma phyllodes

75.1 There is a large bosselated mass in the left breast.

75.2 This is a phyllodes tumour (cystosarcoma phyllodes, serocystic disease of Brodie). This is an uncommon lesion which can occur at any age but which usually affects women aged 30–40 years.

75.3 The patient should undergo mammography and FNA/Tru–cut biopsy of the lesion.

75.4 The majority of tumours are benign. However, some have a stroma which has a high mitotic rate and these may metastasise via blood to lung and bone.

75.5 Treatment requires a wide local excision with a margin of normal tissue around the specimen. Very large benign tumours and malignant tumours are best treated by simple mastectomy.

Endocrine

Case 76 – Carcinoid syndrome

76.1 These facies are characteristic of the carcinoid syndrome.

76.2 Other modes of presentation include: abdominal symptoms – pain, diarrhoea and borborygmi; cardiac disease – pulmonary and tricuspid stenosis or heart failure; dermatological – pellagra; respiratory – asthma.

76.3 The diagnosis of carcinoid tumour is confirmed by measurement of 24 hour urinary 5-hydroxy-indoleacetic acid (5HIAA), a metabolite of serotonin. The syndrome may be diagnosed in the presence of liver metastases which may be detected by ultrasound or CT examination of the liver.

76.4 Carcinoid syndrome arises when a carcinoid tumour, usually ileum or appendix in origin, metastasises to the liver. The serotonin, prostaglandins and kinins which are characteristic of the primary tumour are initially degraded as they pass through the portal circulation. In the presence of liver metastases, these substances are released into the systemic circulation.

76.5 Figure 76b demonstrates an ileal primary with its characteristic appearance, and Figure 76c demonstrates liver metastases which give rise to the syndrome. The primary tumour should be treated by *en bloc* resection regardless of its size since tumour progression and recurrence is often slow. The hepatic metastases can be treated by either local or segmental resection. Another option is hepatic artery embolisation using either inert materials or chemotherapy. Another surgical option which appears beneficial in selected cases is liver transplantation. There are also non-operative options such as treatment with interferon, somatostatin, serotonin antagonists (methysergide maleate) or chemotherapeutic agents (streptozotocin and 5-fluorouracil).

Case 77 – Graves' disease

77.1 She has marked exophthalmos and a diffusely enlarged goitre suggesting a diagnosis of Graves' disease (primary hyperthyroidism).

77.2 The typical biochemical features of Graves' disease are an elevation of both total and free T4 and T3 together with a reduction in TSH. There are also high levels of thyroid autoantibodies.

77.3 There are erythematous plaques of thickened skin, pretibial myxoedema, which is due to deposition of a mucin-like substance in the skin.

77.4 A cardiac history should be taken and an electrocardiogram should be performed since patients with Graves' disease may report angina or have evidence of a sinus tachycardia, atrial fibrillation or heart failure. These patients require beta blockade pre-operatively. All patients undergoing thyroid surgery should also undergo indirect laryngoscopy to check the function of their vocal cords.

77.5 Treatment may be non-operative (anti-thyroid agents or radioiodine) or operative. Anti-thyroid drugs (e.g. propylthiouracil and carbimazole) have an incidence of side-effects including blood dyscrasias; the recurrence rate is high on discontinuing therapy. Radioiodine therapy involves radiation exposure, has a high incidence of hypothyroidism (50% at 10 years), may require several treatments to render the patient euthyroid and is contra-indicated in pregnancy and the young. Surgical treatment attains control rapidly, it avoids the risks of the other two modalities and 95% of patients remain euthyroid at 5 years. There is a small chance of operative damage to the recurrent laryngeal nerve (<1%), hypoparathyroidism (<1%) and hypothyroidism (<5% at 5 years).

Case 78 – Multinodular goitre

78.1 The radiograph demonstrates deviation of the trachea to the left due to the presence of a goitre.

78.2 Other presenting features include: dysphagia, hoarseness or symptoms of hyperthyroidism.

78.3 This is a CT of the thoracic inlet demonstrating a large mass within the right lobe of the thyroid gland extending into the superior mediastinum and obstructing the trachea.

78.4 The aetiology of simple goitres is related to iodine deficiency which may be endemic (Pennines, Alps) or to the ingestion of large amounts of goitrogens such as cabbage. Multinodular goitres usually develop over a period of many years from simple goitres. The nodules represent the result of abnormal thyroid metabolism in which hyperplasia results in hyperplastic nodule formation. Some undergo involution and become filled with colloid whilst others may undergo cystic degeneration or necrosis. 1% of long-standing goitres are said to develop a malignancy.

78.5 The patient has undergone a subtotal thyroidectomy and there are nodules of varying size some of which are cystic and others are filled with colloid. There are also intervening areas of fibrosis. The appearances are typical of a multinodular goitre.

Case 79 – Thyroid carcinoma

79.1 There is a large mass arising from the right side of the neck. The rapid growth together with hoarseness suggest the diagnosis of a malignant thyroid neoplasm.

79.2 The most common malignant thyroid neoplasm is papillary carcinoma (60–65%) which has a 4:1 female:male ratio, affects the young and middle aged, is often multifocal and spreads via the lymphatic system. Follicular carcinoma which represents 15–20% of thyroid neoplasms has a female:male ratio of 3:1 and an average age at presentation of 50 years. This tumour characteristically metastasises haematogenously to the lungs and bones. Medullary carcinomas (5–10%) arise from C cells and may be familial with or without features of multiple endocrine neoplasia. Anaplastic tumours (5–10%) are undifferentiated tumours that occur in older patients and invade local structures.

79.3 A fine needle aspiration is being performed in Figure 79b. Figure 79c is a cytological smear and demonstrates features typical of a papillary neoplasm. FNA cytology has been shown to be reliable in the diagnosis of papillary, medullary and anaplastic carcinomas but is unable to differentiate follicular adenoma from carcinoma since the diagnosis depends upon the histological confirmation of vascular and capsular invasion.

79.4 The management of papillary carcinoma is controversial. The two options are (1) total thyroidectomy, and (2) lobectomy and isthmusectomy. Patients with lymph node metastases should have block dissection of the neck. All patients should receive thyroxine post-operatively. Follicular carcinoma is treated by total thyroidectomy; radioiodine is given to those patients with metastases. Medullary thyroid carcinoma is treated by total thyroidectomy and block dissection of the neck when lymph node metastases are present. Curative surgery is not usually possible for anaplastic carcinoma. Treatment is limited to palliative radiotherapy or isthmusectomy/tracheostomy to relieve dyspnoea.

79.5 Patients with papillary carcinoma have a full life expectancy if disease is confined to the thyroid and 85% 5-year survival with extrathyroidal disease. The prognosis of follicular carcinoma depends on the microscopic invasion of the tumours. Minimally invasive follicular carcinoma has a 97% 5-year survival whereas frankly invasive has a 50% 5-year survival. The prognosis of medullary carcinoma is good in node negative (85% 5-year) but poor in node positive (45% 5-year). There is no 5-year survival in patients with anaplastic tumours.

Case 80 – Primary hyperparathyroidism

80.1 The probable diagnosis is primary hyperpathyroidism. The classical symptoms are 'Bones, stones, abdominal groans and psychic moans'. There is an increased incidence of both urinary calculi and gallstones. There are several causes of abdominal pain including: pancreatitis, peptic ulceration and constipation. The psychiatric component of the disease is depression.

80.2 This investigation is a thallium technetium subtraction scan. The thallium identifies thyroid and parathyroid tissue whilst the technetium identifies thyroid tissue only. Subtracting one image from the other identifies the parathyroids. This scan shows an adenoma of the left upper parathyroid.

80.3 By far the most common pathology is a single parathyroid adenoma (85%) followed by diffuse hyperplasia (11%), multiple adenomata (3%) and carcinoma (<1%).

80.4 Important operation-related complications include recurrent laryngeal nerve palsy (transient in 3% and permanent in <1%) and hypocalcaemia (transient in 40% and permanent in 3%). The cure rate for experienced endocrine surgeons is 95% on first operation.

80.5 This operative picture demonstrates a parathyroid gland which has been stained blue with methylene blue lying alongside the external carotid artery. This is a useful aid in re-operative parathyroid surgery.

Case 81 – Phaeochromocytoma

81.1 The elevated levels of vanillylmandelic acid (VMA), metanephrines and catecholamines are typical of a phaeochromocytoma.

81.2 This is an iodine-131-meta-iodobenzylguanidine (MIBG) scan. MIBG is a radionucleotide that specifically binds to catecholamine precursors and this scan reveals a large tumour in the right adrenal gland.

81.3 Patients undergoing surgery for a phaeochromocytoma should receive pre-operative α-blockade (phenoxybenzamine) and β-blockade (propranolol). Per-operatively, manipulation of the tumour may lead to a 500-fold increase in plasma catecholamine secretion. The tumour should be handled as little as possible until the adrenal veins have been ligated and divided.

81.4 The pathology specimen illustrates the characteristic golden-coloured adrenal tumour.

81.5 Other surgically correctable causes of hypertension include Cushing's syndrome, hyperaldosteronism (Conn's syndrome), coarctation of the aorta and renal artery stenosis.

Case 82 – Cushing's syndrome

82.1 This patient shows features of truncal obesity, striae and multiple ecchymoses. The appearances are typical of Cushing's syndrome. Other features of this condition (not illustrated) include muscle wasting and weakness.

82.2 Cushing's disease as originally described by Harvey Cushing was caused by an adenoma of the pituitary. Causes of Cushing's syndrome include: iatrogenic e.g. corticosteroid treatment; adrenal cortical adenoma or carcinoma; bilateral adrenal hyperplasia; adrenocorticotropic hormone (ACTH) excess or ectopic ACTH production (e.g. squamous carcinoma of lung).

82.3 The diagnosis may be confirmed by estimation of plasma electrolytes, the typical features being hypokalaemia and hypochloraemia. Furthermore, there is elevation of the plasma 17 hydroxycorticosteroid levels.

82.4 This abdominal CT at the level of the adrenal glands demonstrates an adenoma of the left adrenal gland.

82.5 The treatment of choice is surgical excision of the tumour which may be performed by open or laparoscopic routes.

Head and neck

Case 83 – Mixed parotid tumour

83.1 The differential for a lesion in this region includes parotid swellings, sebaceous cysts, lipomas and lymph nodes. Causes of parotid enlargement include primary neoplasms, secondary lymph nodes, infections – viral (e.g. mumps) or bacterial (e.g. post-operative), recurrent swellings (e.g. salivary calculi), chronic parotitis, Sjögren's syndrome and Mikulicz's syndrome. In this case there is a well-defined mass in the parotid gland and should be regarded as a neoplasm until proved otherwise.

83.2 90% of parotid gland neoplasms arise from salivary tissue of which 90% are benign adenomas and 90% lie within the superficial lobe. 75% of these are pleomorphic and are firm with a well-defined border and an irregular surface. These lesions require careful excision as they recur locally if incompletely excised. They carry a small risk of malignant transformation. Adenolymphoma or Warthin's tumours are softer, more mobile and slower growing and are more commonly seen in middle-aged men. They are easier to remove, do not recur locally and rarely undergo malignant change. Neoplasms of intermediate malignancy are acinar cell and mucoepidermoid tumours and the malignant tumours are adenocarcinoma and adenoid cystic carcinoma. The parotid may be affected by non-salivary tumours, e.g. lymphoma.

83.3 A fine needle aspiration will confirm the diagnosis without risk of tumour seeding.

83.4 The treatment of a benign swelling is superficial parotidectomy with removal of tumour without disruption of the capsule. Operation-specific complications include facial nerve palsy through damage of the 7th cranial nerve, parotid duct fistula, haemorrhage and Frey's syndrome (gustatory sweating) – sweating and flushing in the skin innervated by the auriculotemporal nerve during meals. It is believed to be due to cut postganglionic parasympathetic fibres from the otic ganglion regenerating with sympathetics from the superior cervical ganglion and usually develops 6–9 months after the parotid surgery.

83.5 This patient has a large swelling in the left parotid region and on attempting to smile is exhibiting a left facial nerve palsy. The likely diagnosis is a malignant tumour of the parotid.

Case 84 – Submandibular swelling

84.1 An obstructing submandibular duct calculus. The differential diagnosis includes submandibular abscess and lymphadenopathy.

84.2 This is a submandibular sialogram and clearly demonstrates a calculus obstructing the duct.

84.3 Calculi may present at any age and equally in males and females. The majority of salivary gland calculi are associated with the submandibular gland (85%). The predilection of the submandibular gland to develop calculi is related to the higher calcium concentration in saliva from this gland compared to the parotid or sublingual glands.

84.4 A small proportion of stones may be removed per-orally by incising the opening of Wharton's duct and milking the stone along the course of the duct. Most stones will require excision of the submandibular gland, performed through a cervical incision.

84.5 Important structures at risk include the lingual and hypoglossal nerves and the mandibular branch of the facial nerve.

Case 85 – Cervical lymphadenopathy

85.1 The differential includes lymph nodes, thyroid or salivary gland swellings, branchial cysts, sternomastoid tumour, cervical rib, cystic hygroma, aneurysm or arteriovenous fistula, carotid body tumour and cervicofacial actinomycosis.

85.2 Acute inflammation (infection of face, gums, teeth and pharynx), chronic inflammation (e.g. tuberculosis), primary neoplasms (lymphoma), secondary neoplasms, systemic disease (lymphatic leukaemia, syphilis, amyloidosis, infectious mononucleosis, rubella, Still's disease, sarcoidosis, toxoplasmosis).

85.3 A complete examination of the head and neck should be performed including manual inspection and palpation, and mirror examination of oral cavity, tonsillar region, nasopharynx, hypopharynx, piriform sinuses and larynx. Indirect laryngoscopy should then be performed if no cause has been identified.

85.4 Fine needle aspiration (FNA) cytology of the node. If a lymphoma is diagnosed an excisional biopsy is required to obtain further histological information. If the FNA is inadequate, it should be repeated and if still non-diagnostic an open biopsy should be performed. If a carcinoma is diagnosed and the primary tumour not yet identified, endoscopy and bronchoscopy should be performed.

85.5 Tuberculosis.

Case 86 – Thyroglossal cyst

86.1 Thyroglossal cyst.

86.2 Thyroglossal cysts occur as a result of failure of normal obliteration of the migratory tract of the thyroid. Cysts may be identified anywhere along the thyroglossal duct from the lingual foramen cecum to the thyroid isthmus; the majority are infrahyoid.

86.3 Other developmental anomalies sharing a similar aetiology include: lingual thyroid; thyroglossal fistula; thyroid pyramidal lobe; and mediastinal thyroid tissue.

86.4 A radioiodine uptake scan should be performed since the cyst may contain some or all of the thyroid tissue. If the thyroid is located within the cyst then the cyst should be excised and the thyroid tissue isolated and autotransplanted to the neck.

86.5 The operation of choice is excision of the cyst in continuity with the tract and body of the hyoid. If the hyoid is left *in situ* there is a high incidence of recurrence since the cyst traverses the hyoid.

Case 87 – Branchial cyst/sinus

87.1 Branchial cyst.

87.2 Branchial cysts are congenital abnormalities which represent incomplete obliteration of the branchial clefts, usually 1st or 2nd and occasionally the 3rd cleft.

87.3 An important long-term complication is secondary infection which may develop into an abscess. The abscess may then rupture and result in a branchial fistula.

87.4 The cyst should be excised in continuity with its tract. The second cleft runs from the tonsillar fossa through the bifurcation of the carotid artery whilst the first originates at the external auditory meatus and courses in close proximity to the facial nerve.

87.5 This is a branchial fistula or sinus which is termed primary if present from birth or secondary if following discharge of a cyst to the skin.

Vascular

Case 88 – Abdominal aortic aneurysm

88.1 Figure 88a shows an 8 cm abdominal aortic aneurysm on plain abdominal radiography. Figures 88b and 88c are ultrasound images in the antero-posterior and transverse planes from the same patient. Figure 88d is a contrast-enhanced CT scan on the same patient showing extensive thrombus formation in the aneurysm wall. Figure 88e is a per-operative photograph following grafting with a Dacron bifurcation graft.

88.2 The risk factors for the development of aortic aneurysms are male gender, age over 60, cigarette smoking, hypertension, chronic obstructive airways disease, other vascular disease (peripheral, coronary artery, carotid artery) and connective tissue disorders (Marfan's syndrome, Ehlers–Danlos syndrome, pseudoxanthoma elastica).

88.3 The complications of aneurysms are rupture, arterial occlusion, embolisation, fistulation (aortocaval or aortoenteric fistula), infection, chronic consumptive coagulopathy, obstruction of adjacent organs (usually inflammatory aneurysms) – duodenum, ureter. The most common of these complications is aneurysm rupture.

88.4 The size of the aneurysm is the most important factor in determining the risk of rupture. For aneurysms 4.0–6.0 cm in diameter the risk of death from rupture is around 5% per annum. For aneurysms greater than 6.0 cm in diameter the risk is around 15% per annum.

88.5 The mortality from the surgery is around 5%. This is due primarily to associated vascular disease (coronary artery, cerebrovascular, renovascular). Complications are bleeding (from the suture line), infection, aortoenteric fistula, false aneurysms at the suture lines, spinal ischaemia and colonic ischaemia (due to an inadequate collateral circulation from the marginal artery).

Case 89 – Venous ulceration

89.1 Venous ulceration.

89.2 80% of leg ulcers are of venous origin. The differential diagnosis includes arterial ulcer (10%), mixed arterial and venous ulcer, diabetes mellitus, sickle cell disease and vasculitis.

89.3 Venous ulcers arise because of valvular incompetence of the deep or superficial veins. In general incompetence of the former results in a more severe protracted form of ulceration compared with that associated with superficial venous incompetence. It almost always follows deep venous thrombosis. Such thrombotic episodes may be sub-clinical and are commonly associated with pregnancy or following surgery.

89.4 The mainstay of treatment of venous ulceration is compression bandaging, in this instance being achieved by the Charing Cross four-layer bandage. The compression bandaging is changed weekly.

89.5 Figures 89d and 89e show varicose eczema. This is treated by topical application of an emollient cream. More severe cases may be treated by the topical application of a low dose corticosteroid preparation such as betamethasone 0.025%.

Case 90 – Carotid endarterectomy

90.1 Carotid endarterectomy.

90.2 The indications for surgery are symptoms from a 70% or greater stenosis of the internal carotid artery. These symptoms are transient ischaemic attack (including amaurosis fugax), retinal infarction, cerebrovascular accident (patients who make a full recovery or have a permanent but stable neurological deficit). The rationale for operating on these patients is that untreated these patients have a 25% risk of completed stroke over the subsequent 5 years.

90.3 Duplex scanning of the carotid arteries. Carotid arteriography which has as a complication stroke in 1% of patients is no longer a routine investigation.

90.4 The operation is undertaken through an incision along the anterior border of sternomastoid. The controversies in carotid surgery are whether or not one shunts per-operatively (as shown in the illustration) and whether or not one patch closes the arteriotomy.

90.5 The main complications are death (from either stroke or myocardial infarction) and stroke. The combined stroke and death rate should be less than 5%. Other complications include haematoma formation, cranial nerve palsies (VII, IX, X, XI, XII) and wound infection.

Case 91 – Raynaud's syndrome

91.1 Raynaud's syndrome.

91.2 The classical episode affecting the hands/fingers or feet/toes following cold exposure or emotional stimulus is a colour change sequence from white (pallor from vasospasm) through blue (peripheral cyanosis) to red (reperfusion hyperaemia). A large number of patients develop only pallor or cyanosis during attacks. A typical attack lasts between 15–45 minutes.

91.3 The condition most frequently affects females (up to 90%) below the age of 30 years. There is a high prevalence among certain occupational groups, notably those operating vibrating machinery (chainsaw operators, miners, road workers) and those occupations subject to chronic cold exposure (food handlers).

91.4 Up to 50% of patients have an associated disorder, connective tissue disorders (especially scleroderma) being the most common. Other conditions include occlusive arterial disease (atherosclerosis, Buerger's disease, thoracic outlet syndrome, carpal tunnel syndrome) and immunological abnormalities (cryoglobulins, cold agglutinins). The disease tends to be more severe in patients with predisposing conditions compared to those with primary Raynaud's disease.

91.5 The treatment depends upon the severity of the disease. For patients with mild disease appropriate treatment such as cold avoidance, avoidance of cigarette smoking, and wearing thick woollen or electrically heated gloves during the winter months may suffice. Patients engaged in occupations involving cold exposure may not see a resolution of their symptoms until their occupation is changed. Ergotamine preparations and beta-blockers should be avoided. More severe disease may require either medical or surgical intervention. The former includes calcium antagonists (nifedipine), prostaglandin preparations (usually given intravenously) for those with digital ischaemia, and topical nitrates (GTN). Surgical treatment comprises sympathectomy. For the upper limb this may be performed by an open procedure or thoracoscopically. Lumbar sympathectomy for lower limb symptoms can be achieved by an open procedure, laparoscopically or chemically by phenol injection.

Case 92 – Varicose veins

92.1 Varicose veins. The most likely underlying disorder is isolated incompetence of the saphenofemoral junction.

92.2 Patients should be questioned regarding their history of deep venous thrombosis. Patients with a history of deep venous thrombosis may have non-patent deep veins and may thus be relying on the superficial venous system for lower limb venous drainage. Operation in this setting will result in severe oedema and possibly venous gangrene of the affected limb. Such patients should have either a venogram or a Duplex scan of the deep veins to confirm their patency.

92.3 The indication for surgery in most patients is cosmesis, i.e. operation to abolish the unsightly appearance of the dilated veins. Other indications are pain (the veins may ache following periods of standing), superficial thrombophlebitis, bleeding, eczema and ulceration.

92.4 Standard treatment comprises:

1 ligation and division of the saphenofemoral junction at the groin;

2 stripping of the long saphenous vein to knee level;

3 ligation and division of the saphenous vein tributaries at the groin;

4 multiple avulsions of long saphenous varicosities below knee level.

92.5 Complications of surgery are saphenous nerve injury (it is to avoid this complication that the stripper is passed only to knee level), passage of the stripper into a deep vein and inadvertent removal of a deep vein (this is avoided by passing the stripper in a proximal-to-distal fashion), and recurrence of the varicose veins. Recurrence most often results from a failure to ligate and divide all saphenous vein tributaries or the overlooking of a second part of a double long saphenous system. Patients undergoing re-do procedures should have the course of the vein mapped out pre-operatively using Duplex scanning.

Case 93 – Carotid body tumour

93.1 Carotid body tumour (paraganglioma).

93.2 The most common presenting feature is that of a painless palpable lump in the neck. Less commonly symptoms result from cranial nerve (usually vagus and hypoglossal nerves) compression or local infiltration (resulting in dysphagia, hoarseness of voice, stridor or weakness of tongue musculature).

93.3 The differential diagnosis includes a branchial cyst, aneurysm of the common or internal carotid artery, benign and malignant lymphadenopathy.

93.4 Carotid body tumours may be seen at any age, but most commonly patients are between the ages of 40–60 years. Males and females are affected equally. The incidence is greater in those living at high altitudes suggesting that chronic hypoxia may lead to hyperplasia of the carotid body and thence neoplasia. 90% of tumours are considered sporadic; in this setting the incidence of bilaterality is low (5%). Approximately 10% of patients have a familial basis for the condition (autosomal dominant); in this setting the incidence of bilaterality is higher (30%).

93.5 For most patients the appropriate treatment is surgical excision. In the elderly conservative management may be appropriate and for tumours that are unresectable radiotherapy. The tumour is shelled out by creating a plane between it and the blood vessel adventitia. If there is deeper involvement of the carotid artery excision *en bloc* with a cuff of artery may be necessary coupled with patch closure of the carotid artery.

Case 94 – Common femoral artery and popliteal artery aneurysms

94.1 Figure 94a shows a patient who has previously undergone a left above knee amputation. There is a vertical scar from a previous arterial reconstructive procedure and a false aneurysm of the common femoral artery. False aneurysms occur either at the site of an arterial anastomosis or at the site of arterial puncture (penetrating injury, femoral artery catheterisation for arteriography, intravenous drug abusers). They are more common than true aneurysms. Most follow arterial puncture for coronary arteriography.

94.2 Figure 94b is a per-operative photograph of a true aneurysm of the common femoral artery. The aetiology of these is atherosclerosis.

94.3 Figure 94c shows an arteriogram of a popliteal artery aneurysm. Figure 94d shows the appearance of the popliteal fossa following popliteal aneurysm rupture. As with true femoral artery aneurysms the aetiology of these is atherosclerosis.

94.4 Many true femoral artery aneurysms and popliteal artery aneurysms come to light as incidental findings during the course of investigation for other aneurysmal disease. 80–85% of patients with femoral or popliteal artery aneurysms have associated aneurysms of the aortoiliac segments. 70% of true femoral artery and 50% of popliteal artery aneurysms are bilateral.

94.5 The chief complication of popliteal and femoral artery aneurysms is thrombosis and embolism. This may be associated with significant distal ischaemia. Surgical repair is therefore recommended.

Case 95 – Pulmonary embolism

95.1 A radioisotope ventilation–perfusion scan of the lung (V/Q scan) showing multiple non-perfused segments indicating multiple pulmonary emboli.

95.2 Plain chest radiography is usually normal in pulmonary embolism. In a small percentage (5–10%) of patients there may be evidence of pulmonary hypoperfusion evidenced by decreased vascular markings (Westermark's sign). Pulmonary infarction may be seen as a peripheral wedge-shaped opacity or there may be a pleural effusion. Electrocardiographic (except sinus tachycardia) changes are uncommon, but include rhythm abnormalities (atrial fibrillation, heart block) and signs of right heart strain (right axis deviation, right bundle branch block, peaked P-waves in lead II, S-T segment depression and T-wave inversion in the right precordial leads, aVF and lead III). The classic S1 (S-wave in lead I) Q3 T3 (Q-wave and inverted T-wave in lead III) is found in only 5%.

95.3 Predisposing factors include age >40 years, bedrest and immobility, post-surgical states (especially lower limb and abdominal surgery), post-partum state, pelvic and lower limb fractures, congestive cardiac failure, malignancy especially disseminated disease, use of oestrogen-containing oral contraceptives.

95.4 Treatment of established pulmonary embolism is primarily medical. It comprises:

1 thrombolysis with either tissue plasminogen activator or streptokinase;

2 anticoagulation, initially with intravenous heparin followed by conversion to oral warfarin.

The timing of symptoms in relation to surgery will determine whether or not thrombolytic agents can be used. Surgery within the preceding week is a relative contra-indication. The surgical treatment of pulmonary embolism is pulmonary embolectomy, although it is rarely used. Indications for surgery are persistent haemodynamic instability despite adequate resuscitation in a patient with a proven diagnosis of pulmonary embolism.

95.5 Prophylaxis of thromboembolic disease for patients undergoing major surgery is by compression stockings, subcutaneous heparin (5000 IU 8–12 hourly) starting prior to surgery, per-operative use of a pneumatic compression device and early mobilisation.

Case 96 – Diabetes mellitus

96.1 Diabetes mellitus.

96.2 The principal abnormality underlying this is the diabetic neuropathy, possibly compounded by a macroangiopathy and a microangiopathy. The loss of normal sensation results in an incorrect pattern of weight-bearing and ischaemic necrosis over pressure points of the foot. Ulceration and necrotising infection may ensue.

96.3 The principles of treatment are drainage of infection and radical debridement of any necrotic material, if necessary excising ligament, tendon and bone. Close monitoring of the blood glucose and intravenous antibacterials are the other requirements. Broad spectrum antibacterials should be given to cover polymicrobial infections. Gram-positive bacteria are the most commonly implicated, but with more severe infections Gram-negatives and anaerobes are commonly seen.

96.4 Hyperglycaemia should be normalised pre-operatively. Diabetic patients should be placed first on the operative list. They should be starved from midnight. Non-insulin dependent diabetics should omit oral hypoglycaemics on the day of surgery (i.e. discontinued 24 hours preop). Insulin-dependent diabetics should omit medium-acting and long-acting insulin on the day of the operation. Insulin-dependent diabetics require a combination of insulin and dextrose, the dose of insulin administered varying according to the capillary blood glucose on BM stix (sliding-scale insulin).

96.5 Corticosteroids.

Case 97 – Suprainguinal occlusive disease

97.1 Aortograms showing left common iliac artery occlusion (Figure 97a), bilateral common iliac artery stenoses (Figure 97b) and radiograph showing angioplasty balloon *in situ* (Figure 97c).

97.2 The usual presenting feature of aortoiliac atherosclerosis is intermittent claudication of the lower limbs. In general this affects the muscle groups of the buttock, thigh and calves. Over 50% of patients with aortoiliac disease have atherosclerosis of the infrainguinal vessels. These patients tend to have more severe symptoms often presenting with features of critical ischaemia.

97.3 Leriche's syndrome is atherosclerotic occlusion of the aortic bifurcation, typically affecting middle-aged males. The features comprise pallor, symmetrical atrophy and low exercise tolerance affecting both lower limbs in conjunction with impotence.

97.4 The treatment of aortoiliac disease is by:

1   surgery;

2   interventional radiology.

The surgical treatment is reconstruction with aortofemoral bypass grafting. For high-risk patients an extra-anatomic bypass such as axillobifemoral bypass grafting may be used. The trend now is to use radiological techniques. Depending upon the anatomical distribution of the atherosclerosis percutaneous transluminal angioplasty is appropriate for short (<5 cm) subtotal stenoses; following angioplasty a stent is commonly employed.

97.5 Atherosclerosis is a widespread disease. The majority of these patients have significant vascular disease affecting other sites (coronary arteries, cerebral arteries, carotid arteries); the mortality from ischaemic heart disease is high in this patient group. This is the rationale for the administration of anti-platelet agents to these patients. Other measures include cessation of cigarette smoking and the control of hyperlipidaemia, hypertension or diabetes mellitus.

Case 98 – Infrainguinal occlusive disease

98.1 Figure 98a: Arteriogram showing occlusion of the right superficial femoral artery. In addition the patient has undergone a left femoro-popliteal bypass using autogenous saphenous vein.

Figure 98b: Femoro-popliteal bypass using a PTFE graft.

Figure 98c: Polytetrafluouroethylene (PTFE) arterial graft.

98.2 The main symptoms are intermittent claudication (affecting the calf muscles), rest pain and gangrene. Critical ischaemia is defined by one or more of the following criteria:

1 persistent rest pain for a minimum of 2 weeks;

2 ulceration;

3 gangrene in conjunction with an ankle systolic blood pressure of less than 50 mm Hg.

98.3 The ankle-brachial index is the ratio of the systolic blood pressure at the ankle (the higher pressure of dorsalis pedis and posterior tibial arteries) compared to that recorded at the cubital fossa (brachial artery). It is an indication of the degree of lower limb perfusion. The normal value is in the region of 1.0–1.2, claudicants typically have values in the range 0.6–0.9, patients with rest pain in the range 0.3–0.6 and those with impending gangrene <0.3.

98.4 The best long-term patency rates for femoro-popliteal bypass are achieved with the use of autogenous long saphenous vein. The graft may be used in one of two ways. The long saphenous vein may be dissected out, removed and used as a reversed vein graft. Alternatively the vein can be left *in situ*; with this technique all tributaries must be identified and ligated to prevent the creation of arteriovenous communications. The advantage of *in situ* bypass is that the blood supply of the vein is preserved and there is congruity in the size of the anastomoses, i.e. the widest segment of vein is anastomosed to the widest segment of artery (superficial femoral) and the smallest diameter vein end anastomosed to the smallest diameter artery (popliteal or crural). The disadvantage of *in situ* bypass has been mentioned (AV communications).

98.5 If it is not possible to use the long saphenous vein alternative conduits include short saphenous vein, cephalic or basilic vein, PTFE and glutaraldehyde-tanned human umbilical vein graft. The disadvantage of the latter is its expense and its propensity to develop aneurysmal dilatation (for this reason the graft is externally reinforced with a Dacron mesh).

Case 99 – Arterial embolism

99.1 Embolic disease.

Figure 99a: inadvertent intra-arterial injection in an intra-venous drug user resulting in embolism of injected material to the digital arteries of the upper limb.

Figure 99b: neglected brachial artery embolus.

Figure 99c: arteriogram showing brachial artery embolus.

Figure 99d: embolus from a popliteal aneurysm resulting in digital infarction.

Figure 99e: emboli from abdominal aortic aneurysm resulting in 'trash foot'.

99.2 The presenting features of emboli resulting in acute limb ischaemia are the six 'P's: pain, pallor, pulselessness, paraesthesia, paralysis and perishing cold.

99.3 Arterial emboli most commonly arise from the following sites:

1   heart (left ventricular mural thrombus following acute myocardial infarction and in congestive cardiac failure, the left atrium in atrial fibrillation);

2   peripheral blood vessels (aortic or popliteal aneurysm, iliofemoral stenoses).

99.4 The chief differential diagnosis is that of thrombosis of an already atherosclerotic segment of artery. The distinction can sometimes be made on the basis of acuteness of onset of symptoms, but for the lower limb it is often difficult to make the distinction.

99.5 The treatment of embolic disease is medical (thrombolysis) or surgical (embolectomy). There has been a trend away from embolectomy over the last decade or so. Thrombolysis (either with streptokinase or tissue plasminogen activator) is generally given intra-arterially immediately following angiography. The choice between the two therapies depends upon the degree of ischaemia. Patients who have developed paraesthesiae or paralysis of the affected limb should proceed to embolectomy as there may be a significant delay to reperfusion when the time taken for arteriography and thrombolysis is taken into account.

Case 100 – Haemodialysis access

100.1 A side-to-side arteriovenous fistula (Brescia–Cimino) is being constructed between the radial artery and cephalic vein.

100.2 The early complications include: haemorrhage, graft thrombosis, acute left ventricular failure and infection.

100.3 Haemodialysis can also be performed through temporary or permanent central lines which are usually placed into the jugular venous system. Alternatively if vascular access is poor or the patient chooses so, continuous ambulatory peritoneal dialysis can be performed.

100.4 This patient has developed venous hypertension in his left arm. This is usually related to the effects of increased venous flow generating turbulence at points of narrowing (e.g. previous central lines). This subsequently leads to thrombosis and occlusion of flow.

100.5 This patient has developed a false aneurysm at one of his needling sites. This should be repaired and the fistula reinforced with non-absorbable mesh.

Paediatric

Case 101 – Cystic hygroma

101.1 Cystic hygroma.

101.2 The diagnostic feature of cystic hygromas is that they transilluminate.

101.3 Cystic hygromas are hamartomas arising from jugular lymphatics.

101.4 Excision of all cystic tissue is the aim of surgery; however their anatomical location often makes this process difficult.

101.5 Cystic hygromas may enlarge rapidly due to intra-cystic haemorrhage. This may then lead to secondary infection or to the compression symptoms of dysphagia or dyspnoea.

Case 102 – Umbilical hernia

102.1 Umbilical hernia.

102.2 Umbilical hernias are seen in up to 20% of newborns and appear during the first few days of life. They become prominent during crying episodes. Umbilical hernias are seen with increased frequency in babies with hypothyroidism.

102.3 The underlying defect is a weakness of the abdominal wall at the point of insertion of the umbilicus.

102.4 No. The neck of these hernias is large and the risk of strangulation is thus low. Most disappear by 12–18 months and an operation is only considered in those persisting beyond 24 months.

102.5 This is an umbilical polyp, a benign condition that presents with umbilical discharge. The condition usually resolves spontaneously. Simple excision may be required in the face of repeated infections.

Case 103 – Exomphalos and gastroschisis

103.1 Figure 103a is exomphalos and Figure 103b is gastroschisis.

103.2 Exomphalos occurs when there is failure of rotation and re-entry of the herniated midgut during foetal development whereas gastroschisis is a full-thickness abdominal wall defect in which there is herniation of uncovered bowel loops.

103.3 An exomphalos is covered with a sac consisting of foetal membranes and the umbilical cord inserts centrally over the defect. A gastroschisis is not covered by a sac and the herniation invariably occurs to the right of the umbilical cord.

103.4 In both cases the viscera should be kept warm and moist with warm, damp gauze and then packed in a plastic drape to avoid evaporation. The aim in both cases is to return the viscera to the abdominal cavity. The urgency is greatest for gastroschisis since there is no covering membrane and thus there are increased risks of dehydration and sepsis. If the abdominal cavity cannot contain the viscera a polypropylene mesh or silastic tower may be utilised with gradual closure of the abdomen over a period of days.

103.5 Exomphalos has a high incidence (50%) of associated anomalies: skeletal, cardiac, neurological, genitourinary, chromosomal and gastrointestinal (malrotation, Meckel's diverticulum and intestinal atresia). Gastroschisis is rarely associated with other anomalies, but there is a 10–15% incidence of atresias secondary to pressure ischaemia at the neck of the defect. The overall outcome depends on the presence and severity of associated abnormalities.

Case 104 – Diaphragmatic hernia

104.1 The radiograph shows multiple loops of bowel in the left hemithorax and mediastinal shift, diagnostic of a diaphragmatic hernia.

104.2 The infant would appear cyanotic with signs of severe respiratory distress. Percussion of the left chest would reveal a dull percussion note. Auscultation would reveal absent breath sounds in the left hemithorax and possibly bowel sounds.

104.3 The underlying defect is usually a defect of the foramen of Bochdalek and less commonly a defect in the foramen of Morgagni.

104.4 The baby should be resuscitated and undergo a laparotomy with reduction of the hernia and repair of diaphragmatic defect.

104.5 The prognosis depends on the maturity of the lungs and the presence of additional abnormalities (cardiovascular, central nervous system abnormalities and chromosomal defects – trisomy 13 + 18) which are seen in up to 25%.

Case 105 – Pyloric stenosis

105.1 Congenital hypertrophic pyloric stenosis.

105.2 Pyloric stenosis classically affects the first born male and there is a strong familial tendency. It usually presents at 6–8 weeks with projectile vomiting, following which the child is eager to re-feed.

105.3 The investigation is a barium meal and demonstrates a dilated and rotated stomach with failure of barium to pass through the pylorus into the duodenum.

105.4 The classic biochemical picture is of a hypokalaemic, hypochloraemic metabolic alkalosis. This must be corrected prior to surgery.

105.5 This is an operative picture demonstrating a laparoscopic Ramstedt's pyloromyotomy. The muscle has been divided and the mucosa can be seen bulging between the muscle layers.

Case 106 – Intussusception

106.1 This triad of symptoms is classical of intussusception. The most common cause is lymphoid hyperplasia (secondary to an upper respiratory tract infection). Rarer causes include Meckel's diverticulum, intestinal polyps and intestinal duplications.

106.2 This is an ultrasound which demonstrates the doughnut sign which is diagnostic of intussusception.

106.3 This is a barium enema demonstrating an ileocolic intussusception, the most common type of intussusception, with dilated proximal small bowel. In addition to diagnosing the condition, the hydrostatic pressure of the barium may reduce the intussusception in up to 75% of cases.

106.4 This operative picture shows the inner intussusceptum (leading point) and the outer intussuscipiens. The intussusception is reduced and the bowel is examined for both viability and an underlying cause for the intussusception.

106.5 This patient has perioral pigmentation which is typical of Peutz–Jeghers syndrome in which hamartomas are found throughout the small bowel. In addition to acting as a lead point for an intussusception they may cause obstruction or be the source of unexplained abdominal pain or bleeding.

Case 107 – Oesophageal atresia and imperforate anus

107.1 The nasogastric tube is impacted in the oesophagus and cannot be advanced into the stomach. This is characteristic of oesophageal atresia. The most common tracheo-oesophageal anomaly (85% of cases) is a distal tracheo-oesophageal fistula.

107.2 This is a gastrografin swallow which demonstrates an H-type tracheo-oesophageal fistula – 3% of cases.

107.3 If a fistula is present it should be divided. In the case of an atresia, the oesophagus is mobilised to allow an end-to-end anastomosis between two segments of non-atretic oesophagus. If the neonate is unwell or the atretic segment is too long the procedure may be staged with gastrostomy followed by ligation of fistula and oesophageal anastomosis or replacement with a segment of colon or jejunum.

107.4 This is an imperforate anus (anorectal anomaly). The presence of these two conditions should alert one to the possibility of VACTERL syndrome (**V**ertebral, **A**norectal, **T**racheo-**E**sophageal, **R**enal and **L**imb abnormalities).

107.5 High anorectal anomalies require colostomy formation initially, with creation of an anal opening and restoration of bowel continuity as a staged procedure. Low anomalies respond to simple dilatation, with anoplasty in selected patients.

Case 108 – Duodenal atresia

108.1 This X-ray shows the 'double-bubble' which is diagnostic of duodenal atresia.

108.2 Intestinal atresias arise following localised interruptions of the intestinal blood supply during embryonic development.

108.3 There are five subtypes of atresia:

I: muscular continuity with complete web

II: fibrous cord with intact mesentery

IIIa: discontinuous muscle and mesentery

IIIb: apple-peel deformity

IV: multiple atresias

108.4 20–40% of patients with duodenal atresia will have Down's syndrome and its associated features including congenital heart disease.

108.5 A laparotomy is being performed and the atretic segment can be seen. Continuity is restored by performing either a duodeno-duodenostomy with bypass of the atretic segment or duodenojejunostomy with excision of the atresia.

Case 109 – Necrotising enterocolitis

109.1 The neonate has marked abdominal distension with a ladder appearance typical of small bowel obstruction.

109.2 The differential diagnosis of neonatal intestinal obstruction includes: malrotation, volvulus, Ladd's bands, meconium ileus, intestinal atresia, necrotising enterocolitis, annular pancreas, Hirschsprung's disease, small left colon syndrome and imperforate anus.

109.3 There is gas within the intestinal wall. In a neonate this is typical of necrotising enterocolitis (NEC).

109.4 NEC occurs as a result of intestinal mucosal injury and thus the pathogenesis is multifactorial and includes: infection – *Clostridium*, *Pseudomonas aeruginosa*, *Enterobacter cloacae*, *Staphylococcus aureus*; ischaemia – decreased cardiac output, hypoxaemia, acidosis, hypothermia, hyperviscosity; hyperosmolar feeding. These factors lead to both local effects (oedema, microvascular thrombosis, luminal distension with decreased intramural blood flow, transmural necrosis and perforation) and systemic effects (bacterial translocation, endotoxin and exotoxin release, cytokine activation, multi-organ dysfunction).

109.5 Between 50 and 90% of patients can be managed non-operatively with aggressive resuscitation, nasogastric decompression, antibiotic therapy and parenteral nutrition. Surgery is limited to patients in whom there is evidence of perforation or refractory/recurrent septic episodes. The principles of surgery are excision of non-viable bowel and exteriorisation of the bowel. Multiple enterostomies may be required. Overall survival is 60–70% with outcome dependent on associated anomalies.

Case 110 – Wilms' tumour

110.1 The important differentials for an abdominal mass in childhood are: kidney – nephroblastoma (Wilms' tumour), autosomal recessive polycystic kidney disease; neuroblastoma; liver – hepatoblastoma, hepatocellular carcinoma, haemangiona; spleen.

110.2 This is an intravenous urogram and demonstrates distortion of the left pelvi-calyceal system.

110.3 The CT demonstrates bilateral Wilms' tumours, the left being larger than the right. Approximately 6% of patients have bilateral tumours at the time of presentation.

110.4 The inferior vena cava must be imaged by USS/CT for evidence of invasion and the liver and lungs as both organs are common sites for metastases.

110.5 The recognised treatment for Wilms' tumour is surgical excision and chemotherapy (vincristine and actinomycin-D). Favourable prognostic indicators include young age, early tumour stage and a well-differentiated tumour. A favourable tumour has a cure rate of up to 90% but the cure rate falls to 50% in the presence of metastases. The patient shown (see Figure 110b) underwent left nephrectomy and partial right nephrectomy combined with chemotherapy.

Case 111 – Undescended testis

111.1   The differential diagnosis lies between retractile testis, undescended testis, testicular agenesis and testicular hypoplasia. The most likely diagnosis is undescended testis.

111.2   A retractile testis occurs secondary to overactivity of the cremaster muscle and the testis can be manipulated back into the scrotum by gentle manipulation in a warm atmosphere. An undescended testis however cannot be manipulated into the scrotum. The other conditions require imaging to confirm the diagnosis.

111.3   Use of ultrasound, CT or MRI may help to localise the testis prior to operation.

111.4   An undescended testis may occur anywhere from the abdomen to the apex of the scrotum and requires orchidopexy.

111.5   Long-term sequelae of undescended testes include: defective spermatogenesis (sterility if bilateral); torsion; trauma; inguinal herniation is associated in up to 90%; malignancy, with a relative risk of 20–40%.

Case 112 – Ectopic testis

112.1   There is an oval mass in the perineum and an empty left hemiscrotum suggesting a diagnosis of ectopic left testis.

112.2   Ectopic testes occur when following normal descent through the inguinal canal, the testes become trapped in a pocket between Scarpa's fascia and the external oblique fascia.

112.3   Ectopic testes may also found in the superficial inguinal pouch, at the base of the penis and in the femoral triangle.

112.4   Yes – unlike undescended testes.

112.5   The testis is explored and orchidopexy performed.

Case 113 – Phimosis

113.1 There is a pin-hole opening in the foreskin with scarring of the tissues surrounding the aperture. This is a phimosis.

113.2 Phimosis is a fibrous contraction of the preputial aperture which makes it impossible to retract the foreskin. As a consequence there is ballooning of the foreskin and a build up of smegma leading to recurrent episodes of balanitis.

113.3 Circumcision.

113.4 Religious circumcision, cosmetic, paraphimosis.

113.5 This patient demonstrates preputial adhesions. These may be broken down with a blunt probe following the application of a local anaesthetic cream.

Case 114 – Torsion

114.1 Torsion of testis, torsion of hydatid of Morgagni, testicular tumour or epdidymo-orchitis.

114.2 The testis has been explored and found to be necrotic.

114.3 Recognised predisposing factors include: undescended testis; horizontal testis; high investment of tunica vaginalis.

114.4 Emergency surgery is mandatory since after 6 hours irreversible testicular ischaemia occurs. The scrotum is incised and the testis delivered. If it is black it is either necrotic or ischaemic. It should be untorted and wrapped in a moist, warm swab to observe whether or not it recovers. If the testis is not viable an orchidectomy should be performed. If viable an orchidopexy should be performed. It is important to fix the contralateral testis as the predisposing anatomic anomaly occurs bilaterally.

114.5 This is a torted appendix testis (hydatid of Morgagni) which should be excised.

Case 115 – Inguinal hernia

115.1 Indirect inguinal hernia.

115.2 In children the male to female ratio is about 9:1 with prevalence being age-related (highest among pre-term infants). 5% of inguinal hernias in children are diagnosed in the neonatal period, 30% are diagnosed during the first year and the remaining 65% during childhood.

115.3 The underlying defect in all cases is a patent processus vaginalis and thus all indirect hernias result from a congenital defect. The abdominal contents enter the canal following repeated stretching of the deep ring and may then progress along the inguinal canal and into the scrotum.

115.4 Yes. All children, with inguinal herniae should undergo an operation since the hernial defect is often small and thus the risk of strangulation is high.

115.5 The cord contents have been carefully isolated and a herniotomy is being performed.

Urology

Case 116 – Transitional cell carcinoma of the bladder

116.1 Ultrasound scan of the bladder (Figure 116a) showing a papillary tumour and a pathological specimen (Figure 116b) of a transitional cell carcinoma.

116.2 Painless haematuria is the presenting feature in over 80% of patients. Frequency, dysuria and urgency are seen in 20%. Other presenting features include loin pain secondary to ureteric obstruction, recurrent urinary tract infections or microscopic haematuria.

116.3 Intravenous urogram and cystoscopy.

116.4 Transitional cell carcinoma was first noted to be associated with certain occupations (aniline-dye, rubber, paint, chemical industries) that involved exposure to aromatic hydrocarbons (benzidine, naphthylamine). Other factors are cigarette smoking, chronic ingestion of analgesics (phenacetin), cyclophosphamide therapy and prior radiotherapy to the pelvis.

116.5 At presentation 75% of bladder cancers are superficial, i.e. superficial to the muscularis layer and can be managed by transurethral resection and intravesical therapy alone. The remainder of cancers are invasive and in these transurethral therapy is insufficient. In the absence of distant metastases radical therapy in the form of radiotherapy or cystectomy is required. The former is current practice in the UK and the latter in the US.

Case 117 – Renal cell carcinoma

117.1 Contrasted CT scan showing a renal cell carcinoma of the right kidney (Figure 117a). Figure 117b shows the typical macroscopic appearance of such a tumour.

117.2 The most common presenting features are haematuria, loin pain and the presence of a palpable abdominal mass. Other features include systemic features (fever, malaise, weight loss), hypertension, nausea and vomiting. Up to one-third of patients have features of a para-neoplastic syndrome. These include anaemia or polycythaemia (due to erythropoietin secretion), hypercalcaemia (due to PTH-related peptide secretion), raised erythrocyte sedimentation rate, coagulopathies, deranged liver function tests, neuropathies and myopathies.

117.3 In the absence of distant metastases treatment is by radical nephrectomy (*en bloc* removal of the kidney, adrenal and perinephric fat in their envelope of Gerota's fascia; the proximal ureter and the renal vascular pedicle). Approximately 5% of renal cell carcinomas are associated with direct tumour extension into the inferior vena cava, and possibly the right atrium. In these cases thrombectomy is combined with the nephrectomy. For the infradiaphragmatic portion of the IVC this can be achieved by venotomy and repair. For supradiaphragmatic tumour extension cardiopulmonary bypass will be necessary to effect tumour removal.

117.4 Chest radiograph showing solitary 'cannonball' pulmonary metastasis. Long-term survival following resection of these metastases is not uncommon. Renal cell carcinomas and testicular teratomas show a propensity for the development of solitary pulmonary metastases.

117.5 Angiomyolipoma.

Case 118 – Germ cell tumour of the testis

118.1 Germ cell tumour of the testis, in this case seminoma.

118.2 The usual presenting feature is a scrotal mass or scrotal pain. In a small proportion of patients tumour-secreted hormones result in gynaecomastia, reduced libido or infertility.

118.3 Probably not. Classical seminomas (40%) produce neither alpha-foetoprotein or beta-human chorionic gonadotrophin, the tumour markers used commonly to monitor testicular germ cell tumours. Two-thirds of testicular tumours are composed of one tumour element. The remainder are composed of more than one element; thus a proportion of patients with seminomas may produce hormonal products by virtue of the heterogenous nature of the lesion.

118.4 Orchidectomy should be performed through an inguinal incision with early clamping of the spermatic cord vessels to prevent possible tumour dissemination during mobilisation of the testis. The spermatic cord is ligated at the internal inguinal ring and the testis and cord structures below the internal ring removed. If there is evidence of extratesticular disease (15%) on staging CT, radiochemotherapy is given in addition. All regimens used contain cisplatin as a chemotherapeutic agent.

118.5 The most common testicular tumours in males over the age of 50 are non-Hodgkin's B-cell lymphomas. They are usually associated with disseminated disease.

Case 119 – Benign prostatic hyperplasia

119.1 Figure 119a is a transrectal ultrasound scan of the prostate showing a small adenoma. It is possible to take either a fine-needle aspirate for cytology or a Tru-cut biopsy of the prostate under ultrasound guidance, if a mass lesion is seen.

119.2 A flow-rate study and an ultrasound abdomen to measure post-micturition residual bladder volume. In general assuming a voided volume of 200 ml or greater, a maximum urinary flow rate of less than 10 ml/s is highly suggestive of obstruction. A residual volume of greater than 100 ml suggests chronic retention of urine. Given the symptoms these findings would be indications for surgery.

119.3 A resectoscope (Figure 119b) and prostatic chippings (Figure 119c) obtained at the time of transurethral resection.

119.4 The complications of TURP are urinary tract infection, haemorrhage, clot retention, failure to void following catheter removal, urethral stricture, incontinence, retrograde ejaculation and impotence. A rare complication is the transurethral syndrome, thought to be due to absorption of the irrigation fluid. The result is fluid overload and hyponatraemia. The condition manifests as hypotension, bradycardia, confusion, nausea and in severe cases, convulsions. Treatment is by intravenous infusion of 2M saline solution combined with frusemide.

119.5 Invariably patients with long-term indwelling urinary catheters have bacterial colonisation of the bladder urine. They are thus at greater risk of peri-operative urinary tract infection. Prophylactic antibacterials should be given at the time of the operation and continued post-operatively. The antibacterial should have activity against Gram-negative bacteria.

Case 120 – Adenocarcinoma of the prostate

120.1 Adenocarcinoma of the prostate.

120.2 A plain film of the pelvis (Figure 120a) and lumbar spine (Figure 120b) showing the classic sclerotic type of metastasis associated with carcinoma of the prostate. This is confirmed by the radio-isotope bone scan showing 'hot-spots' of isotope uptake corresponding to these sites (Figures 120c and 120d).

120.3 No. This depends upon the state of his general health. If debilitated by the malignancy, insertion of a urinary catheter and palliation may be the treatment of choice. Otherwise an operation is indicated on the grounds of bladder outflow obstruction (TURP). This would also provide tissue for a histologic confirmation of the diagnosis.

120.4 The treatment of this condition is divided into the treatment of local (prostatic) disease and the treatment of disseminated disease. Tailoring treatment will involve staging of the disease with prostate-specific antigen level (levels <20 ng/ml bone metastases rare, levels >100 ng/ml bone metastases inevitable), CT scanning and isotope bone scanning (in those with a PSA >20 ng/ml). The treatment of local disease is either radical radiotherapy or radical prostatectomy. The treatment of disseminated disease utilises the hormonal dependence of prostatic tissue. The aim is to produce castrate levels of androgens. Methods used include bilateral orchidectomy, oestrogens (diethylstilboestrol), luteinising hormone-releasing hormone analogues (buserelin, goserelin, leuprorelin, triptorelin) or antiandrogens (flutamide, cyproterone acetate).

120.5 Prostate cancer is the third most common cause of cancer death in the Western World. The incidence of the disease increases with increasing age; it is rarely seen below the age of 50 years. The median age at diagnosis is 72 years. A high incidence is seen in North America and Western Europe and a low incidence in Asia. In the US the incidence in black males is 1.5–2.0 times that of white males. It is unknown in males castrated before puberty. The first-degree male relatives of index patients have an eight-fold greater risk of developing prostate cancer.

Case 121 – Hydrocoele

121.1 No.

121.2 To determine the nature of a scrotal swelling one must be able to answer the following: can one palpate above the swelling? Can the testis and epididymis be palpated? Does the swelling transilluminate?

121.3 A hydrocoele.

121.4 The treatment depends upon the age of the patient and whether or not the patient wishes to have any treatment. An infantile hydrocoele results from a patent processus vaginalis and in most cases it resolves spontaneously by the end of the first year. If it is still present at this time operation is indicated; management is as for an infantile inguinal hernia and comprises ligation of the patent processus. For adult hydrocoeles aspiration of the fluid is the simplest method of treatment although the fluid generally reaccumulates. Surgical excision is by one of two methods: Jaboulay procedure (excision of redundant tunica vaginalis and eversion) and Lord's procedure (plication of the tunica).

121.5 The main complication of any scrotal surgery is haematoma formation. The elastic nature of the scrotal skin and fascia enable the development of a haematoma with only minimal tamponading effect.

Case 122 – Calculous disease of the urinary tract

122.1 Figure 122a is a plain abdominal film and Figure 122b, a delayed intravenous urogram film, taken at 24 hours. The latter shows no excretion from the right urinary tract because the contrast passed rapidly through on the previous day. There is an obstructing calculus at the left pelviureteric junction with the left kidney imaged as a tomogram. A ureteric stent has been inserted (Figure 122c) to allow drainage of the left kidney in order to preserve functioning renal tissue.

122.2 This stone is best managed by percutaneous nephrolithotomy. In the absence of obstruction the stone could be managed by extracorporeal shock wave lithotripsy.

122.3 Eighty per cent of urinary calculi are composed of calcium oxalate, 15% are triple phosphate stones (calcium magnesium ammonium phosphate), and 5% uric acid stones. Cystine stones account for less than 1%.

122.4 The condition primarily affects males (M:F 3:1) between the ages of 30–50 years. The lifetime risk of developing urinary calculi is 2–3%. There is approximately a 50% risk of recurrent stones within the next ten years. First-degree relatives of patients with stone disease are at greater risk of developing the condition themselves.

122.5 Predisposing medical conditions act by altering the urinary excretion of calcium, cystine, oxalate or uric acid. These include disorders of calcium metabolism (hyperparathyroidism, renal tubular acidosis), increased oxalate absorption (following terminal ileal resection in Crohn's disease), disordered uric acid metabolism (gout) and disordered cystine metabolism (cystinuria).

Case 123 – Varicocoele

123.1 Varicocoele.

123.2 The left side is affected 98% of the time.

123.3 The condition usually affects young adults.

123.4 Usually a varicocoele is asymptomatic save the patient's awareness of a collection of dilated veins ('bag of worms') in their scrotum. It may cause a dragging or aching sensation in the scrotum, and has been reported to be associated with infertility. The latter is supposed to result from a defective countercurrent thermal exchange mechanism between the testicular artery and pampiniform plexus of veins resulting in a higher intratesticular temperature, at which spermatogenesis occurs suboptimally.

123.5 When indicated, surgical treatment comprises ligation and division of the internal spermatic veins (the continuation of the pampiniform plexus). This is achieved through either an inguinal or an abdominal approach. The latter may be performed laparoscopically.

Case 124 – Transitional cell carcinoma of the ureter

124.1 A retrograde (or ascending) urogram. The radiograph is obtained by cannulating the ureteric orifice at the time of cystoscopy and injecting contrast medium. An intravenous urogram will image the same region.

124.2 It shows a filling defect in the middle third of the right ureter, most likely to be a transitional cell carcinoma.

124.3 Tumours of the renal pelvis and ureter account for only 5% of urothelial cancer. Transitional cell carcinoma constitutes 90% of these tumours, and squamous cell carcinomas the remainder. The tumour occurs most commonly in males (M:F 3:1) between the ages of 50–70 years. The ratio of bladder:renal pelvis:ureter urothelial tumours is 50:3:1. There is a high incidence of the condition in parts of Bulgaria, Romania and Yugoslavia where it is associated with endemic Balkan nephropathy.

124.4 Treatment depends upon the general health of the patient, the presence of distant metastases and the amount of functioning renal tissue on the affected side. In general the treatment for proximal tumours is a nephroureterectomy and for distal tumours a distal ureterectomy with reimplantation of the ureter into the bladder.

124.5 Urothelial cancer is a 'field disease' with a tendency for multifocality; thus the main risk to the patient is of metachronous urothelial cancer. Approximately 30% of patients with upper tract transitional cell carcinomas develop bladder cancer. The more proximal in the urinary tract the tumour the greater is the risk of subsequent disease. Around 50% of those with upper ureteral tumours will develop lower ureteral tumours subsequently, whereas only a small proportion of those with lower ureteric tumours subsequently develop upper ureteral tumours.

Case 125 – Adult polycystic kidney disease

125.1 Adult polycystic kidney disease.

125.2 Autosomal dominant inheritance, the gene being located on chromosome 16. If you cannot recall whether a disease is inherited as an autosomal dominant or recessive trait, remember that recessively inherited conditions are generally enzyme deficiencies that result in a severe disorder early in life with many index cases not surviving to reproduce. Autosomal dominant conditions on the other hand are less severe and thus index cases survive into the reproductive years. If the clinical manifestations do not appear until beyond the second decade of life the disease is thus likely to be dominantly inherited.

125.3 Features of the condition are gross enlargement of both kidneys (weight can be up to several kg) and replacement of the substance by cysts. Cysts may be found in the liver (30%), spleen (15%), and pancreas (10%). Associated features are berry aneurysms of the circle of Willis, hypertension, features of chronic renal failure, polycythaemia, valvular heart disease and abdominal wall hernias.

125.4 The condition does not usually become evident (except family member screened patients) until the fourth decade when it presents with loin pain and/or haematuria as a result of haemorrhage into a cyst, abdominal discomfort due to gross organomegaly and local pressure effects, hypertension or symptoms of chronic renal failure. Increasingly, relatives of affected individuals are diagnosed at a pre-clinical stage by ultrasound imaging of the kidneys (starting at the end of the second decade).

125.5 It is the most common inherited disorder leading to renal failure, accounting for approximately 10% of patients receiving renal replacement therapy. A proportion of these patients will undergo renal transplantation.

Case 126 – Fournier's gangrene

126.1 Fournier's gangrene.

126.2 It results from a synergistic infection between anaerobic and aerobic bacteria.

126.3 Treatment comprises intravenous antibacterials (aerobic and anaerobic cover) and surgical debridement of the affected tissue. Depending upon the size of the defect it can be left either to heal by granulation or tissue cover obtained (split-skin grafts or pedicled skin flap from the thigh/lower abdomen).

126.4 The original description of the condition by Fournier in 1883 was of a spontaneously occurring infection in previously fit, healthy young males in the absence of any predisposing factors. Most cases seen now have a predisposing factor such as recent perineal surgery, urinary catheterisation, ongoing urinary tract or intra-abdominal sepsis. A high proportion of these patients are diabetic.

126.5 Figure 126b shows necrotising fasciitis of the right upper limb. Necrotising fasciitis of the abdominal wall, usually following surgery, is known as Meleney's gangrene.

Case 127 – Renal transplant

127.1 The early post-operative complications include acute tubular necrosis, renal artery thrombosis, renal vein thrombosis, acute rejection, ureteric obstruction, urinary leak, urinary tract infection and immunosuppressive-induced nephrotoxicity.

127.2 Figures 127a and 127b demonstrate gum hypertrophy and hirsutism both of which are recognised complications of cyclosporin immunosuppression.

127.3 Figure 127c is an arteriogram demonstrating a stenosis of the transplanted renal artery close to its junction with the native external iliac artery. Figure 127d demonstrates the results of balloon angioplasty on the stenosis.

127.4 The CT demonstrates a mass of para-aortic lymph nodes which are compressing the inferior vena cava. This is a non-Hodgkin's lymphoma. The lymphomas are usually B-cell in origin and are believed to be related to Epstein–Barr virus infection.

127.5 At one year the expected graft and patient survival are 90% and 95% respectively.

Orthopaedics and trauma

Case 128 – Dislocation of the shoulder and elbow

128.1 Anterior dislocation of the shoulder (Figures 128a, 128b) and dislocation of the elbow (Figure 128c).

128.2 Treatment is reduction of the dislocation under intravenous sedation. For the shoulder several methods are employed. They include:

1 traction with counter-traction;

2 Kocher's method;

3 Hippocratic method;

4 gravitational traction. This is useful in children.

Failure to achieve reduction by these methods is an indication for reduction under general anaesthesia. Reduction of an elbow dislocation is by forearm traction whilst progressively flexing the elbow.

128.3 Early complications are:

1 neurological injury: shoulder – axillary nerve, suprascapular nerve or posterior cord of brachial plexus; elbow – median or ulnar nerve. Always test nerve function prior to attempting reduction and document this clearly in the patient's case notes;

2 arterial injury: shoulder – axillary artery; elbow – brachial artery;

3 associated fractures.

128.4 Late complications include joint stiffness and recurrent dislocation. A particular problem encountered with elbow injuries is myositis ossificans. Prevention of this complication is the proposed basis for the encouragement of active mobilisation of the elbow joint following injury and the avoidance of passive mobilisation.

128.5 Posterior dislocation of the shoulder and luxatio erecta. These are uncommon. The former is associated with involuntary muscle contractions such as those seen during epileptic seizures and following electric shocks. Luxatio erecta, the rarest form of shoulder dislocation, occurs with the arm held in full abduction.

Case 129 – Fracture of the clavicle and surgical neck of humerus

129.1 Fracture of the right clavicle at the junction of the medial 2/3 and the lateral 1/3 in a child (Figure 129a) and an adult (Figure 129b). Figure 129c shows a fracture of the surgical neck of the humerus.

129.2 Early complications are rare, but include neurovascular injury or pneumothorax. Late complications are malunion and non-union. Fractures of the lateral third are those most likely to give rise to a non-union. A degree of malunion is inevitable and occurs because of an inability to completely support the weight of the upper limb during fracture healing. In children this generally remodels to leave a good cosmetic result, but in adults it is not uncommon for a lump to remain.

129.3 The fracture should be treated with a broad arm sling for 2–3 weeks until pain permits mobilisation. Fractures associated with significant displacement (usually lateral third fractures) should be treated operatively.

129.4 The most widely used classification is that by Neer which subdivides the fractures according to the involvement of the humeral head, humeral shaft, lesser tuberosity and greater tuberosity.

129.5 Treatment depends upon the fracture classification. In general Neer types I–III can be treated conservatively in a sling until pain subsides (2 weeks), then pendulum movements until active movements are commenced when fracture healing has occurred (6 weeks). Neer types IV and V should be treated by reconstitution of the fragments using a cancellous screw to secure the tuberosities to the humeral head. Neer types VI are treated by dislocation reduction and then according to the guidelines as for the remainder. Severely displaced three fragment and four fragment fractures carry a high risk of subsequent avascular necrosis and thus hemi-arthroplasty or total joint replacement should be considered.

Case 130 – Fracture of the ankle

130.1 Radiograph showing a small avulsion fracture of the right medial malleolus following an eversion injury (Figure 130a), clinical photograph (Figure 130b) and radiograph (Figure 130c) of a bimalleolar fracture of the right ankle.

130.2 No. The most common ankle injury is a lateral ligament complex rupture, which may or may not be accompanied by an avulsion fracture of the lateral malleolus. Ligament injuries are treated by strapping of the ankle (tubigrip) and a period of non-weight-bearing on the affected side. More severe ligament injuries (and avulsion fractures) are treated in a below-knee plaster cast for 6 weeks.

130.3 The most common grading of ankle fractures is the Weber classification that revolves around the notion that the fibula is the chief source of ankle stability. Its usefulness is in its assessment of the degree of fracture-associated ankle joint instability.

Type A fracture is below the level of the tibiofibular syndesmosis. The medial malleolus may be fractured and the medial collateral ligament disrupted. Following reduction the ankle is stable.

Type B fracture is an oblique fracture of the fibula where the fracture line runs upwards from the level of the ankle joint. The medial malleolus is usually fractured and the medial collateral ligament disrupted. The syndesmosis is intact and thus the fracture stable upon reduction.

Type C fracture is where the fracture line is above the level of the tibiofibular syndesmosis. The syndesmosis is ruptured, there is diastasis and thus the fracture is unstable. As well as reconstitution of the fragments treatment of the diastasis is necessary.

130.4 The complications of ankle fractures are vascular injury, persistent swelling, reflex sympathetic dystrophy, malunion, joint stiffness and osteoarthritis.

130.5 In this patient achieving wound closure is a major consideration. It is likely to require skin grafting.

Case 131 – Methods of fracture fixation

131.1 Figure 131a: fracture of the left tibia and fibula managed by non-operative means.

Figure 131b: fracture of the left femoral shaft managed by interlocking intramedullary nailing.

Figure 131c: fracture of the right radius and ulna managed by plating.

131.2 The main early local complications of long bone fractures are infection and injury to surrounding structures in particular neighbouring neurovascular bundles. The main late local complications are delayed or non-union, malunion, myositis ossificans and ischaemic contractures. Most systemic complications of long bone fractures occur early; they include adult respiratory distress syndrome, shock and coagulopathy as a result of the fat emboli syndrome, thromboembolic disease, crush syndrome, systemic sepsis from local infection and hypovolaemic shock from blood loss (femoral shaft fractures).

131.3 External fixation (not shown) would be appropriate if there was gross contamination of the fracture site.

131.4 Gustilo's classification of open fractures is used to define the degree of associated tissue damage in an open fracture. It is used to guide treatment and gives a prognosis for the risk of subsequent wound infection. The risk of infection is lowest in type I wound and maximal in type III wounds.

I: Simple fracture with a clean wound less than 1 cm in size.

II: An associated wound of >1 cm in size but without extensive soft-tissue damage.

III: Severe injury associated with extensive soft-tissue damage and local contamination.

IIIA = Open fractures where there is adequate soft-tissue coverage.

IIIB = Open fractures associated with extensive soft tissue loss, periosteal stripping and bone exposure.

IIIC = Open fracture associated with arterial injury.

131.5 Stress fractures are fractures occurring in normal bone of healthy people as a result of bone fatigue due to repetitive exercise. They are seen commonly in long distance runners, military recruits and dancers. Presenting features are pain at the site and localised tenderness. Depending upon the duration of symptoms, plain radiography may be normal (first 3–6 weeks) or may show a small transverse defect in the cortex and a periosteal reaction. The bones most frequently affected are the shafts of the tibia, fibula, femur, humerus, second metatarsal, the pars interarticularis of L5 and the navicular. Treatment is rest, with the main goal of this being prevention of a complete cortical fracture.

Case 132 – Fracture of the femoral neck

132.1 Fracture of the left femoral neck. Figure 132a shows external rotation and shortening of the left leg. Figure 132b is a radiograph of the pelvis showing a subcapital fracture of the left femoral neck.

132.2 The fracture occurs in the elderly, especially females and is associated with post-menopausal osteoporosis. Many follow only trivial trauma. It is much more common in white races compared with black and Asian races.

132.3 The Garden classification.

I: A fracture through one cortex (the upper cortex) associated with impaction

II: A fracture through both cortices with impaction, but no displacement

III: Fracture through both cortices associated with partial displacement of the two fragments

IV: Fracture through both cortices associated with complete displacement of the two fragments

132.4 Complications specific to this fracture are avascular necrosis of the femoral head and non-union. Both are more common in Garden grades III and IV.

132.5 Treatment is directed toward the Garden grade and the general state of the patient. There are three options:

1 closed reduction and internal fixation;

2 hemiarthroplasty (femoral head replacement);

3 total hip replacement.

Younger patients and medically fit elderly patients are managed by closed reduction and internal fixation of the fracture with cannulated screws. Those patients subsequently developing the complications listed above can be converted to a total hip replacement at a later date. Most other patients will be managed by hemiarthroplasty. Occasional medically fit elderly patients with Garden type IV fractures will be managed with a total hip replacement. The disadvantage of performing a total hip replacement for fractured femoral neck is the higher dislocation rate compared with the rate for elective replacement.

Case 133 – Fracture of the femoral neck

133.1 Thompson hemiarthroplasty (Figure 133a), AO cannulated screws (Figure 133b), dynamic hip screw and plate (Figure 133c), intramedullary nail with locking screws (Figure 133d).

133.2 A dynamic hip screw and plate is used for intertrochanteric fractures of the femur. The intramedullary nail is being used to treat a subtrochanteric fracture.

133.3 Some subtrochanteric (the more proximally located) fractures can be treated with a long plate dynamic hip screw. Subtrochanteric fractures are commonly pathological, i.e. through a metastatic deposit.

133.4 Pubic ramus fractures may be a cause of non-weight-bearing in this age group. Examine specifically for point tenderness at these sites. Treatment comprises bed rest and analgesia, mobilising as pain permits.

133.5 Undisplaced intertrochanteric fractures may not show on plain radiography. Thus elderly patients presenting with hip pain and a normal plain film should be admitted for further investigation, either by magnetic resonance imaging or by isotope bone scanning.

Case 134 – Supracondylar fracture of the humerus and fracture of the olecranon

134.1 Supracondylar fracture of the left humerus (Figure 134a) and transverse fracture of the left olecranon (Figture 134c).

134.2 The former has been treated by manipulation under general anaesthetic and Kirschner-wiring (Figure 134b), the latter by tension band wiring (Figure 134d).

134.3 Supracondylar fractures of the humerus are associated with neurovascular injury (brachial artery and median nerve). Brachial artery injury may be associated with the development of a forearm compartment syndrome which if unrecognised may subsequently result in Volkmann's ischaemic contracture. Other complications include malunion resulting in a varus or less commonly a valgus deformity. Considerable time (up to one year) often elapses before there is return of elbow extension. As with all injuries around the elbow joint myositis ossificans may occur.

134.4 Olecranon fractures by their nature are intra-articular and thus predispose to osteoarthritis in the elbow joint.

135.5 The signs of a forearm compartment syndrome are disproportionate pain despite what would be considered a standard dose of analgesia, pain on passive extension of the fingers, sensory loss, altered distal pulses, swelling and tenderness of the forearm. Treatment is removal of all constricting bandaging, plaster casts and careful observation. If symptoms do not settle a fasciotomy should be undertaken. The wound is then re-inspected 5–7 days later and either closed primarily if feasible, skin grafted or left to close secondarily. Compartment pressure can be measured; however, the diagnosis is a clinical one and if a normal compartment pressure is recorded but the diagnosis suspected, fasciotomy should be performed.

Case 135 – Fractures around the wrist

135.1 The radiographs are of a right Colles' fracture (Figure 135a), a right Barton's fracture (Figure 135b) and a greenstick fracture of the distal radius (Figure 135c).

135.2 The Colles' fracture should be treated by manipulation under intravenous sedation followed by immobilisation in a plaster cast for 6 weeks. Undisplaced Colles' fracture do not require manipulation. Unstable fractures require plating or treatment with an external fixator.

135.3 This fracture may be confused with a Smith's fracture (reverse Colles' fracture). However, in a Smith's fracture the fracture line is transverse and extra-articular. The fracture line in a Barton's fracture is oblique and intra-articular; associated with the fracture is a subluxation of the carpus with the distal fragment. The fracture is best treated by a buttress plate placed anteriorly.

135.4 Complications of Colles' fracture include malunion, delayed union and non-union; rupture of the extensor pollicis longus tendon and reflex sympathetic dystrophy. The latter is characterised by swelling and tenderness of the finger joints, painful movements and vasomotor signs.

135.5 Greenstick fractures of the distal radius are treated by a Colles' type plaster cast. Immobilisation is for 3 weeks only however. Uncommonly the fracture line may be complete and resemble the typical Colles' fracture seen in adults. The rule of 5s is a guide to the time to union for fractures. For fractures of the upper limb the time to union of cancellous and cortical bone is 5 and 10 weeks respectively. For fractures of the lower limb double these values, i.e. 10 and 20, and for children halve the corresponding values.

Case 136 – Fracture of the carpal scaphoid

136.1 Fracture of the scaphoid bone. Radiography for a suspected scaphoid fracture should include a film in ulnar deviation as the fracture gap is maximised in this view.

136.2 Typically the fracture affects young adults (usually males).

136.3 Tenderness in the anatomical snuffbox. If there is localised tenderness to this point but the initial radiograph is normal, treatment is on clinical grounds by immobilisation in a plaster cast, re-examination and repeat radiographs at 2 weeks. If the radiographs are still normal but there is evidence of persistent tenderness treatment either continues along clinical grounds (6 weeks immobilisation) or further imaging of the carpus is obtained (isotope bone scan, magnetic resonance imaging).

136.4 The most feared complication of this fracture is avascular necrosis of the proximal fragment. The blood supply of the scaphoid enters in a distal-proximal direction; thus fractures through the proximal portion of the bone are likely to result in a disruption of this. As a result the proximal fragment undergoes avascular necrosis, non-union follows and osteoarthritis of the wrist joint ensues.

136.5 Fractures of the scaphoid tubercle require no treatment other than a support dressing and mobilisation as pain permits. Undisplaced fractures are treated in a plaster cast for 6 weeks. If following removal of the cast there is persistent tenderness at the fracture site the cast is re-applied for a further 6 weeks. Continued signs of non-union are treated by bone grafting and insertion of a Herbert compression screw. Displaced fractures are treated in the first instance by open reduction and insertion of a Herbert compression screw.

Case 137 – Spinal injury

137.1 Radiographs showing fracture-subluxation of C5 and fracture-dislocation of the lower thoracic spine.

137.2 The main concern with vertebral column fractures is risk of associated spinal cord injury. Most spinal cord injuries are apparent at the time of the injury; however, significant vertebral column injuries may exist in the absence of neurologic injury and thus the principle of treatment is to prevent any further neurologic damage. Certain injury patterns make the possibility of a spinal cord injury more likely: those with injuries above the level of the clavicle or significant head injuries are at higher risk of cervical spine injury. Any high-energy transfer injuries such as those from high-velocity vehicles or falls from heights increase the risk of spinal injury.

137.3 Yes. A lateral cervical spine radiograph should show the skull base, all seven cervical and the first thoracic vertebrae.

137.4 Four people are required to log-roll a patient with proven or suspected spinal injury. One person is responsible for each of the following:

1 providing manual, in-line immobilisation of the head and neck;

2 turning the trunk (including pelvis and hips);

3 turning the pelvis and legs;

4 directing the log-roll and moving the spinal board.

137.5 Denis's classification subdivides the spine into three columns. The anterior column is composed of the anterior longitudinal ligament, the anterior portion of the intervertebral disc and the anterior two-thirds of the vertebral body. The middle column is composed of the posterior third of the vertebral body, the posterior portion of the intervertebral disc and the posterior longitudinal ligament. The posterior column is composed of the neural arch, the pedicles, the facet joints, the spinous process, the interspinous and the supraspinous ligaments. In general stable injuries are those with disruption of only one column and unstable injuries those with disruption of two or more columns.

Case 138 – Head injury

138.1 Skull radiograph of an occipital fracture (Figure 138a), lateral skull radiograph showing a fracture of the left temporal bone extending into the skull base (Figure 138b). The latter is evidenced by the air-fluid level in the sphenoid sinus. Figure 138c is a CT scan of the head showing a left frontal extradural haematoma.

138.2 The Glasgow Coma Scale. This is a composite scoring system made up of three parameters: eye-opening response, verbal response, motor response. The best response achieved in each category is scored. Grading is as follows:

Eye-opening

  4 spontaneous

  3 to speech

  2 to pain (not facial pain)

  1 no eye-opening

Verbal response

  5 appropriate conversation

  4 confused conversation (but questions answered)

  3 inappropriate words (recognisable words, but no coherence)

  2 incomprehensible sounds (grunts and groans)

  1 no verbal response

Motor response

  6 obeys

  5 localises (changing the location of the pain stimulus causes movement towards the stimulus)

  4 withdrawal (movement away from painful stimulus)

  3 abnormal flexion (decorticate posture)

  2 extensor response (decerebrate posture)

  1 no motor response

A severe head injury is defined as a score of eight or below.

138.3 The indications for hospitalisation following a head injury are confusion/coma, neurologic deficit, skull fracture, patients that are difficult to assess, i.e. those under the influence of alcohol or drugs, the mentally handicapped, patients with coexistent medical morbidity such as haemophilia and patients who do not have a responsible adult at home with them.

138.4 Primary brain injury is that occurring at the time of head injury. Secondary brain injury is that occurring following the initial insult. In general this means maintaining a satisfactory cerebral perfusion pressure and metabolism, i.e. preventing hypoxia, hypotension, hypoglycaemia. Further neurosurgical prevention includes the use of diuretics, judicious use of intravenous fluids and induction of hypocapnia. These measures should not be carried out except under the supervision and direction of a neurosurgeon.

138.5 The danger with all basal skull fractures is infection. Technically, these are compound fractures and thus ascending infection (meningitis, cerebral abscess) may occur, usually with pathogens that colonise the respiratory tract. Patients should be treated prophylactically with appropriate antibacterials.

Case 139 – Burns and inhalation injury

139.1 These patients were caught in a house-fire. They should be managed according to the Advanced Trauma Life Support guidelines (ABC):

Airway with cervical spine control

Breathing and ventilation

Circulation and haemorrhage control

139.2 The three radiographs obtained during the resuscitation process following the primary survey are an anteroposterior chest and pelvis, and a lateral cervical spine.

139.3 The term secondary survey denotes a head-to-toe examination of the trauma patient following the initial (primary) survey and the commencement of resuscitation. It includes a full neurologic examination, rectal (and vaginal) examination, log-rolling of the patient so that the spine and posterior trunk may be examined and the insertion of urinary and nasogastric catheters.

139.4 Yes, they are at high risk of inhalation injury and thus potential airway problem from laryngeal oedema. They have evidence of facial burns and singeing of the eyebrows. Other features suggesting inhalation injury are carbon deposits in the oropharynx, the expectoration of carbon-tinged sputum. Features in the history that make inhalation injury likely are a history of explosion and entrapment in an enclosed burning area. Once laryngeal oedema has occurred intubation may prove difficult. It is thus often easier to ventilate electively in this scenario.

139.5 The rule of nines is a guide to the percentage body surface area affected by burns and thus a guide for fluid replacement regimes. The following body areas account for approximately 9% of the body surface area: head and neck, all of one upper limb, one side of chest, one side of abdomen, one side of one lower limb. The perineum makes up the deficit of 1%. It is useful in adults, but inappropriate in children as the head forms a greater portion of the surface area and the limbs less. The Lund and Browder charts provide a more useful guide in children.

Case 140 – Thoracic trauma

140.1 The photograph (Figure 140a) is of the left upper anterior chest wall showing tyre marks on the skin; the patient has been struck by a vehicle and run over. Figure 140b shows a left tension pneumothorax (there is evidence of medistinal shift) and Figure 140c shows a simple right pneumothorax with evidence of subcutaneous emphysema.

140.2 Tension pneumothorax is a clinical diagnosis and should be treated immediately by needle decompression in the second intercostal space (mid-clavicular line) and then chest drain insertion (anterior axillary line in the 5th intercostal space). One should not wait to confirm the diagnosis radiologically.

140.3 The signs of a tension pneumothorax are profound respiratory distress (tachypnoea, hypoxia, cyanosis), hypotension, tachycardia, distended neck veins, tracheal deviation, hyper-resonant chest percussion and absent breath sounds. Tension pneumothorax results in displacement of the heart and great vessels to the contralateral side. Kinking of the great vessels results in an inadequate venous return to the right atrium and thus an insufficient cardiac output.

140.4 The indications for chest drain insertion in a trauma patient are pneumothorax (simple and tension), massive haemothorax, patients with suspected chest trauma who are going to be intubated and subject to positive pressure ventilation, and patients with suspected chest trauma who are going to be transferred by either air or ground.

140.5 Cardiac tamponade. This is treated by pericardiocentesis and then by thoracotomy.

Case 141 – Abdominal trauma

141.1 The patient has undergone a splenectomy for splenic haematoma following blunt trauma. The ultrasound scan is from a different patient but shows a splenic rupture. Lower left rib fractures are commonly seen in association with splenic injuries.

141.2 The peritoneal lavage catheter is inserted in the midline one-third of the way along a line joining the umbilicus with the symphysis pubis. Warmed Hartmann's solution or normal saline are infused to a total volume of 10 ml/kg (maximum 1 litre). A positive result is the aspiration of frank blood, the presence of 100 000 erythrocytes/ml or more, or the presence of 500 leucocytes/ml or more.

141.3 The indications for diagnostic peritoneal lavage in a trauma patient are:

1   when the examination is hampered by confounding variables such as intoxication with alcohol or drugs, the presence of a head injury or patients that are difficult to assess such as the mentally handicapped and children;

2   when the patient is going to undergo lengthy imaging procedures or general anaesthesia for other injuries;

3   when the examination findings are equivocal due to the presence of other injuries: fractures of the pelvis, lumbar spine and lower ribs.

The pitfalls of peritoneal lavage are the false negatives with retroperitoneal injuries (which are better imaged by CT scanning) and the false positives that may occur with pelvic fractures (in this instance the lavage catheter should be inserted above the umbilicus).

141.4 The other indications for splenectomy are:

1   incidental, at the time of another operation such as gastrectomy;

2   for the treatment of hypersplenism, e.g. myelofibrosis, lymphoproliferative disorders (Hodgkin's disease, chronic lymphocytic leukaemia), Gaucher's disease, splenic vein thrombosis;

3   for the treatment of autoimmune disease, e.g. autoimmune haemolytic anaemia, immune thrombocytopenic purpura;

4   for the treatment of haemolytic anaemia due to red cell abnormalities, e.g. spherocytosis, elliptocytosis;

5   for the treatment of primary splenic cysts and tumours.

141.5 The spleen is a major site of opsonisation, notably for encapsulated bacteria such as *Streptococcus pneumoniae*, *Neisseria meningitidis* and *Haemophilus influenzae*. Splenectomy increases the risk of subsequent infection with these organisms. The syndrome of overwhelming post-splenectomy sepsis (OPSI) typically occurs following a prodrome of an upper respiratory tract infection. Within hours septicaemia may occur. The risk of OPSI is greatest in children, in the first 2 years following splenectomy, those immunosuppressed by concurrent lymphoproliferative disorders and those with thalassaemia. Prophylactic vaccines (pneumococcal, meningococcal, *Haemophilus*) are administered preoperatively to patients undergoing elective splenectomy and post-operatively to trauma patients. In addition, antibacterial prophylaxis with penicillin V is recommended for all patients under the age of 20 undergoing splenectomy and those at high risk of OPSI (listed above).

Case 142 – Osteoarthritis

142.1 Plain radiographs showing a right Charnley total hip replacement *in situ* and left hip osteoarthritis (Figure 142a) and the same patient following left Zimmer CPT total hip replacement (Figure 142b). Joint replacement was performed for osteoarthritis.

142.2 The radiographic features of osteoarthritis are loss of joint space, sclerosis of the subchondral bone, subarticular cysts formation and osteophyte formation. The joints most commonly affected by osteoarthritis are the hip, knee, vertebral column facet joints and the interphalangeal joints of the hands and feet.

142.3 Treatment of osteoarthritis of the hip is divided into non-operative and operative. Non-operative measures include analgesics, physiotherapy and the use of a stick (held on the affected side). The three principal operations for osteoarthritis of any joint are osteotomy, arthrodesis and joint replacement. Indications for operative intervention are worsening pain, in particular features such as associated sleep disturbance, progressive loss of mobility and thus limitation of normal activities. By and large the procedure of choice is a total hip replacement. Certain constraints make this impractical in younger patients. Their life-span far exceeds the anticipated life-span of a prosthetic joint and thus subsequent revision

arthroplasty is likely. In occasional patients realignment femoral osteotomy and arthrodesis are employed.

142.4 The most feared complication of total hip replacement and any joint surgery is infection. The rate should be less than 1%. Prophylactic measures include the use of laminar air flow, antibacterials and the donning by theatre staff of all-in-one complete body gowns that incorporate a visor. Other complications include thromboembolic disease, dislocation (higher with the posterior approach to the hip and in patients undergoing total joint replacement as a primary procedure for fractured neck of femur), heterotopic bone formation around the joint, loosening of one or both of the components, sciatic nerve injury and erosion of the acetabular component into the pelvis.

142.5 Predisposing conditions include:

1 congenital and childhood hip disorders, e.g. congenital dislocation of the hip, Perthe's disease, slipped upper femoral epiphysis;

2 intra-articular fractures;

3 avascular necrosis;

4 septic arthritis;

5 rheumatoid arthritis.